A Patient's Guide to Heart Rhythm Problems

A Johns Hopkins Press Health Book

A Patient's Guide to Heart Rhythm Problems

Todd J. Cohen, M.D., F.A.C.C., F.H.R.S.

The Johns Hopkins University Press

Baltimore

© 2010 Todd J. Cohen
All rights reserved. Published 2010
Printed in the United States of America on acid-free paper
9 8 7 6 5 4 3 2 1

The Johns Hopkins University Press
2715 North Charles Street
Baltimore, Maryland 21218-4363
www.press.jhu.edu

Library of Congress Cataloging-in-Publication Data
Cohen, Todd J.
    A patient's guide to heart rhythm problems / Todd J. Cohen.
        p. cm.
    Includes bibliographical references and index.
    ISBN-13: 978-0-8018-9774-0 (hardcover : alk. paper)
    ISBN-10: 0-8018-9774-2 (hardcover : alk. paper)
    ISBN-13: 978-0-8018-9775-7 (pbk. : alk. paper)
    ISBN-10: 0-8018-9775-0 (pbk. : alk. paper)
    1. Arrhythmia—Popular works. 2. Arrhythmia—Treatment—Popular works. I. Title.
    RC685.A65C558 2010
    616.1'28—dc22   2010007500

A catalog record for this book is available from the British Library.

Figures 1.1, 1.2, 1.3, 8.1, 10.1, and 11.1 are by Jacqueline Shaffer.

Special discounts are available for bulk purchases of this book. For more information, please contact Special Sales at 410-516-6936 or specialsales@press.jhu.edu.

The Johns Hopkins University Press uses environmentally friendly book materials, including recycled text paper that is composed of at least 30 percent post-consumer waste, whenever possible. All of our book papers are acid-free, and our jackets and covers are printed on paper with recycled content.

Contents

Color illustrations follow page 36

Foreword

....

This book is a useful and informative guide for patients and their families dealing with cardiovascular disease and heart rhythm health issues. Even though sudden cardiac arrest is the nation's leading cause of death, it is often misunderstood or confused with other cardiac conditions.

The Sudden Cardiac Arrest Association is dedicated to making patients more aware of sudden cardiac arrest. This awareness includes risk factors, emergency response, prevention, and treatment options. Dr. Todd Cohen shares our passion for making people smarter about their health and their medical care options. That is why we are grateful to him for his efforts in writing this book and doing it in a way that answers and addresses the many questions patients have about sudden cardiac arrest. A family history of heart disease or sudden cardiac death and a personal history of heart disease, smoking, obesity, or diabetes are reasons enough to pay attention to what Dr. Cohen has written.

Use this book as a reference and a guide. Make notes in the margins. Write down questions you want to ask your physician. If your primary care doctor does not have the answers, he or she can refer you to a cardiac specialist who can better address your concerns.

Your heart is an amazing thing. It pumps the blood and oxygen the rest of your body requires for your good health, and it is the symbolic center of the love you have for your family, friends, and everything you hold dear. So read this book to take care of your heart and to take care of those special people in your life.

Chris Chiames, Executive Director
Sudden Cardiac Arrest Association

Preface

....

This book is dedicated to my patients and to everyone with medical problems that need treatment. Various sources of information have been available to you over the years, including magazine articles, pamphlets (often provided by the manufacturers of implantable devices), and information your physician has provided in discussing your condition and treatment. This book is another source of information. It presents basic concepts of how the normal heart functions, and then expands on these concepts to discuss abnormalities in heart rhythms along with the consequences of heart rhythm disturbances. It discusses tests and studies used in diagnosing heart rhythm problems, and finally, it describes treatments and prevention measures.

My intention in this book is to provide background to help patients understand their diagnosis, any tests they may undergo, and how doctors might treat the problem. Illustrations and tables are provided to clarify the concepts.

Always ask questions. There is usually an opportunity before any procedure for your doctor and his or her team to answer all your questions and to make sure you are entirely comfortable before proceeding. What is best for you must be considered individually. It is with all these factors in mind that I wrote this book, as a resource for patients, their families, and their loved ones. I hope it helps you gain further understanding of your condition, and I hope it helps you get better and stay well.

PART ONE

The Basics

CHAPTER 1

Overview

....

Your Heart

Your heart is a muscular structure, located in the middle of your chest, that pumps blood throughout your body. It is a vital organ with both electrical and mechanical components. The electrical system produces a rhythm, and the mechanical components provide the pumping. Mechanically, the heart has four chambers and four valves, as shown in figure 1.1. The heart consists of two upper chambers and two lower chambers. Each upper chamber is called an *atrium* (right atrium and left atrium). Together, these chambers are called the *atria*. They *receive* blood, which is then pumped into the lower chambers. The lower chambers, called the *ventricles* (right ventricle and left ventricle), *pump* blood to the lungs and to the rest of the body.

The electrical system (which is also called the conduction system) tells the heart (and its chambers) when and in what sequence it should contract and relax to pump blood to the rest of the body (figure 1.2). The electrical impulses begin high up in the right atrium, in a structure called the *sinus,* or *sinoatrial, node* (SA node). A node is defined as a beginning structure or a point for electrical signals to come together and then be redirected to another region in the heart. There are two nodes in the heart: the SA node and the AV node. Impulses move from the SA node across the atrial structures to the AV node (located in the middle of the heart, between the atria and ventricles). A small delay in the electrical signal typically occurs in the AV node before the impulse travels to the His bundle;

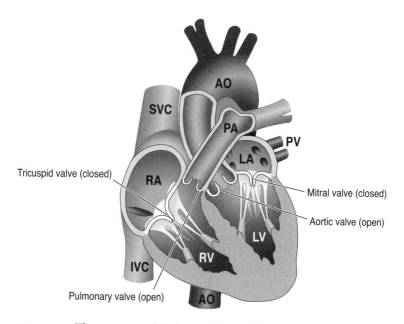

FIGURE 1.1. The structure of the heart—its chambers, valves, and great vessels. AO = aorta, IVC = inferior vena cava, LA = left atrium, LV = left ventricle, PA = pulmonary artery, PV = pulmonary veins, RA = right atrium, RV = right ventricle, SVC = superior vena cava. (See also color version.)

it then moves down through the right and left bundles to specialized Purkinje fibers before activating the ventricles.

The presence of disease in any of the specialized electrical conducting tissues may disrupt the flow of electricity through the heart, slowing or pausing the heart rate. When the heart rate is too slow, a person may develop symptoms and may need to have a pacemaker surgically implanted to correct the problem. Disease inside or outside the specialized cardiac conduction tissue can also result in fast heart rhythm problems that might require treatment with medications, catheter ablation (a procedure that identifies the heart rhythm abnormality and destroys specific tissue to cure the rhythm problem), or an implantable device such as a defibrillator (see part 7).

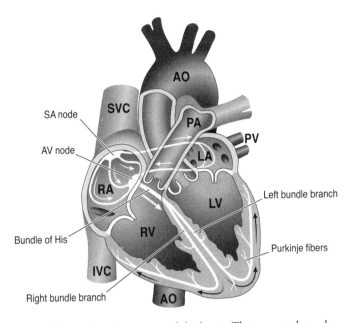

FIGURE 1.2. The conduction system of the heart. The arrows show the electrical impulses, which begin in the sinus node and travel through the atria to the atrioventricular node. After a slight delay there, these impulses are conducted through the His bundle and through the right and left bundle branches to the Purkinje fibers, which carry the impulses into the ventricles. AO = aorta, AV node = atrioventricular node, IVC = inferior vena cava, LA = left atrium, LV = left ventricle, PA = pulmonary artery, PV = pulmonary veins, RA = right atrium, RV = right ventricle, SA node = sinus node, SVC = superior vena cava. (See also color version.)

Blood Movement through the Heart

Blood flow through the heart chambers should be smooth and rhythmic. The right side of the heart receives blood removed of oxygen from the rest of the body via two large veins called the *superior vena cava* and *inferior vena cava* (figure 1.3). Blood enters the right atrium and travels through the tricuspid valve to the right ventricle. Then it is pumped out the pulmonary valve through the pulmonary artery into the lungs, where oxygen is put into the blood. Oxygen-

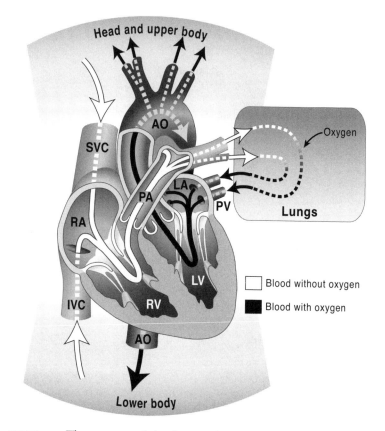

FIGURE 1.3. The sequence of circulation. The white arrows show blood deprived of oxygen (deoxygenated blood) returning to the right side of the heart. The blood is then pumped to the lungs to receive oxygen. Oxygenated blood, indicated by black arrows, returns to the heart via the pulmonary veins and is then pumped from the left side of the heart to the rest of the body. AO = aorta, IVC = inferior vena cava, LA = left atrium, LV = left ventricle, PA = pulmonary artery, PV = pulmonary veins, RA = right atrium, RV = right ventricle, SVC = superior vena cava. (See also color version.)

ated blood returns through pulmonary veins to the left side of the heart, into the left atrium. The blood then travels across the mitral valve into the left ventricle and is pumped out through the aortic valve into the aorta and then to the rest of the body.

TABLE 1.1   *Heart facts*

- The heart is a four-chambered muscular structure.
- It is about the size of your fist but can get much larger with disease.
- It pumps 1,500 gallons of blood each day.
- It normally beats at a rate of 60 to 100 times per minute (your heart rate).
- It beats about 100,000 times per day and 36 million times per year.
- Heart muscle does not usually regenerate.

The heart itself is nourished through the coronary arteries, which arise from the proximal (first part of the) aorta. The coronary arteries consist of a left coronary artery (which branches into the left anterior descending and the left circumflex coronary arteries) and a right coronary artery. Blockages in these arteries (or in their branches) may lead to a lack of blood flow and oxygenation of heart tissue (called *ischemia*). When the blockage is severe and lasts long enough (usually following plaque rupture), the person may have a heart attack (also called a *myocardial infarction*; see chapter 12). For a summary of basic facts about the heart, see table 1.1.

CHAPTER 2

Who Is Your Cardiologist?

A cardiologist is a doctor who specializes in the care of patients who have (or are suspected of having) heart disease. A *general cardiologist* specializes in a wide range of heart-related problems. In addition to medical school training, cardiologists have three years of internal medicine preparation and at least three years in cardiology. Subspecialists such as those described below often have training beyond that of general cardiologists.

A *cardiac imaging cardiologist* specializes in noninvasive imaging studies that help diagnose structural and functional abnormalities of the heart. Studies include echocardiography, computer tomography angiography (CT angiography) with contrast dye, cardiac magnetic resonance imaging (cardiac MRI), and nuclear cardiology (see part 5).

A *cardiac electrophysiologist* specializes in diagnosing and treating heart rhythm problems by invasive and noninvasive means and typically has at least one additional year of training beyond general cardiology training. These cardiologists perform an invasive procedure called an *electrophysiology study* to help diagnose a particular rhythm problem (see chapter 21). Once the rhythm abnormality is identified, it can be treated with a special tube (called a *catheter*) that maps and ablates (gets rid of) the problem (see chapter 23). In addition, these doctors can treat heart rhythm abnormalities with devices such as implantable cardiac monitors, pacemakers, and defibrillators (see part 7).

An *interventional cardiologist* specializes in the diagnosis and treatment of heart-related problems by inserting catheters into blood vessels and then injecting contrast dye into the catheters to visualize abnormalities. One of the invasive procedures these specialists perform is a percutaneous coronary intervention (PCI), in which coronary artery blockages are opened via a balloon (angioplasty), and one or more stents (small metal mesh tubes) are placed to keep the vessels open (see chapter 19). This specialty typically requires one year of additional training beyond general cardiology.

A *cardiac rehabilitation cardiologist* is a general cardiologist who helps patients recover from heart surgery and other heart interventions using a graduated and monitored exercise program. These doctors often educate patients and coach them on healthy diet, exercise, and lifestyle modifications.

A *heart failure specialist* is a cardiologist who specializes in the treatment of congestive heart failure and helps patients maintain an optimal diet and lifestyle. These specialists also prescribe and monitor patients' medications and strive to provide optimal medical therapy (see chapter 33).

A *cardiothoracic surgeon* performs open-heart surgery to bypass blocked arteries and to treat valvular heart disease. The cardiac surgeon may also perform procedures to treat heart rhythm abnormalities and has the advantage of directly visualizing the heart. Cardiothoracic surgery encompasses entirely different surgical training than is required in general cardiology and its subspecialties.

CHAPTER 3

The Pulse
Heartbeat and Rhythm

··

When the heart muscle pumps (or contracts), blood is sent throughout the body via a series of pipes called arteries. The blood carries
oxygen and nutrients to the brain and to the rest of the body's vital
organs and then returns to the heart via a similar series of blood vessels called veins. With each contraction of the heart, the blood being
propelled can be felt as a series of pulsations known as the arterial
pulse. The pulse is basically a reflection of the pumping of blood
from your heart through the arterial blood system throughout the
body. Your heart's pulsation may be felt (or palpated) in various
places, including over the chest near where the heart is located, as
well as at the wrist (radial pulse), the groin (femoral pulse), and the
neck (carotid pulse).

The quality of the pulse and the rate of your heart rhythm can
be measured by taking your pulse. You or a family member should
use the radial pulse location, at the wrist, because this is the most
practical place to feel a pulse consistently. To take your pulse, with
your palm up, place the first and second fingers of your other hand
(do not use your thumb) over the wrist on the thumb side (figure
3.1). This is where your radial pulse can be found. You should be
able to feel the quality of the pulse itself. Is it strong, indicating an
adequate blood pressure (or perfusion)? Or is it weak, indicating a
lack of adequate blood pressure? Is it fast or slow? By counting the
number of pulsations over a fifteen-second interval and multiplying
that number by four, you can calculate your heart rate (in beats

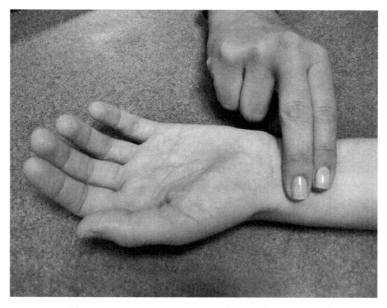

FIGURE 3.1. The proper way to take your pulse. With palm up, place two fingers of your other hand on the thumb side of the wrist to feel the pulse. The heart rate can be calculated by counting the number of palpated beats over 15 seconds and then multiplying that number by 4. For example, if 20 beats are counted over a 15-second period, that number multiplied by 4 gives a heart rate of 80 beats per minute.

per minute). A normal heart rate is between 60 and 100 beats per minute. Pulse facts helpful to cardiac patients and their families and friends are shown in table 3.1.

One of the most significant (and common) problems faced by heart patients is a heart rhythm abnormality. For example, sudden cardiac arrest (see chapter 12) is most often the result of very rapid heart rhythms, called *ventricular tachycardia* or *ventricular fibrillation*, in which the lower chambers of the heart are beating too fast to effectively pump blood to the rest of the body (see chapter 8). If the person loses consciousness, his or her pulse may feel weak or may even be impossible to feel. If the rhythm is not treated immediately or does not revert to a normal or slower rhythm on its

TABLE 3.1   *Pulse facts*

- Take your pulse with your first and second fingers, not your thumb.
- Count the number of heartbeats that occur in 15 seconds and multiply that number by 4 to get the heart rate in beats per minute.
- The normal heart rate is 60 to 100 beats per minute.
- Heart rates slower than 60 beats per minute can be normal if you don't have symptoms such as fatigue, shortness of breath, light-headedness, or dizziness.
- Rapid heart rates (greater than 100 beats per minute) may be normal or abnormal, depending on circumstances.

own, the person will not survive. If, however, the patient is treated immediately with cardiopulmonary resuscitation (CPR; see chapter 37) or advanced cardiac life-support measures, including defibrillation (a shock administered to the chest by means of a defibrillator; see chapter 38), or if the rapid rhythm breaks on its own accord, a palpable pulse may be restored (indicating the return of adequate circulation), and the person will usually survive.

CHAPTER 4

Heart Rhythms

Normal Conduction

The normal heart beats regularly, with typical rates between 60 and 100 beats per minute, and the flow of electrical impulses is sequential, beginning in the SA node (see chapter 1) and traveling through atrial tissue, which causes atrial muscle to contract. Electrical impulses continue through the AV node, His bundle, and Purkinje fibers, and then to the ventricles, causing the muscles in the ventricles to contract. This flow of electrical impulses from atria to ventricles helps to propel blood from the heart to the rest of the body. The cycle typically repeats well over 2 billion times in the course of a lifetime. Disease in the normal conduction system may result in a slow or fast heart rate or an irregular heartbeat. Blocked electrical impulses from the atria to the ventricles are termed *heart block*.

Arrhythmia: Abnormal Heart Rhythms

Problems can occur anywhere in the electrical system and interfere with the pumping mechanism of the heart. In addition, problems can occur outside the conduction system, possibly as a result of disease within the heart muscle itself. Conditions that weaken the heart muscle may cause rapid heart rhythms, called *tachycardias*, with rates greater than 100 beats per minute and possibly much faster. The faster the heart rate, the greater the chance that delivery of oxygen and other nutrients to the brain and other organs will be impaired. With very fast heart rhythms (greater than 200 beats per minute), the person will likely become light-headed and dizzy and even pass out. The heart may also beat too slowly (called *bradycardia*), with heart rates below 60 beats per minute. An irregular heart rate might indicate early beats, called premature contractions (coming from either the atria or the ventricles), or may be an indicator of a rhythm problem called *atrial fibrillation*, in which the atria beats at rates greater than 400 beats per minute.

The heart should beat in a regular rhythmic fashion. An arrhythmia is a heart rhythm that is irregular or in other ways inappropriate; it is not a "normal rhythm." Arrhythmias may be initiated in the atria or in the ventricles. People may or may not have symptoms, such as a pounding heartbeat (fluttering), heaviness in their chest, shortness of breath, sweating, dizziness, passing out, or a feeling of impending doom (feeling of death). Cardiac arrest is the complete collapse of the patient's circulatory system and unfortunately is the first symptom for some people. The different kinds of heart rate abnormalities are discussed further in the chapters that follow. The causes, symptoms, and treatment of various arrhythmias are similar, with slight differences; understanding the differences can be challenging, but for a heart patient, reaching this understanding is important.

CHAPTER 5

The Pump

....

The heart is, in fact, a pump. It receives blood deprived of oxygen; oxygen is added to the blood; and the heart then pumps the blood to the rest of the body. A strong heart muscle and proper timing of the opening and closing of the heart valves ensure adequate delivery of oxygenated blood to the body's vital organs and tissues. Certain heart valves must open at specific times to allow the forward flow of blood and must close at other times to prevent backflow (blood flowing back into the chambers rather than out to the body). The timing of the opening and closing of the valves is controlled by the heart's conduction system. If the valves are incompetent or are unable to handle a large volume of fluid because of ineffective pumping from the heart, fluid will back up and accumulate in the lungs and other tissues, resulting in congestive heart failure, whose symptoms include shortness of breath, leg swelling, and fatigue.

Your doctor may describe the strength of your heart using terms such as cardiac output and ejection fraction. *Cardiac output* is a measure of how much blood your heart can pump out in liters per minute. A normal cardiac output is greater than 4 liters per minute. *Ejection fraction* (EF) is a more commonly used term than cardiac output; it represents the *percentage* of blood that is ejected from the heart. EF can be measured through various imaging modalities, including echocardiography, angiography, and cardiac MRI, or as part of a nuclear study. These studies approximate the EF by calculating the difference between the amount of blood contained within the left ventricle during a full contraction and the volume of blood contained there during a complete relaxation, divided by the amount of blood in a complete relaxation phase; this number is then multiplied by 100 to give the EF as a percentage. A normal EF is greater than 50 percent. A low EF may place you at risk for a life-threatening heart rhythm problem, which may result in sudden loss of consciousness or sudden cardiac arrest and may result in death if not promptly treated. For a summary of key ejection fraction facts, see table 5.1.

First and foremost, every heart patient should know his or her EF. If your EF is 35 percent or less, ask your doctor if you could benefit from an implantable cardioverter defibrillator (ICD). This device is typically implanted in the chest and can detect heart rhythm abnormalities (fast and slow) and treat them accordingly (see chapter 27). The EF table (table 5.2) can help you assess the strength of your heart. A low EF may be associated with signs and symptoms of heart failure (see chapter 33).

TABLE 5.1 *Ejection fraction facts*

- Ejection fraction (EF) measures the percentage of blood that is ejected from the heart.
- The EF can be calculated through various tests by determining the difference between the volume of blood in the left ventricle at the end of a full contraction and the volume of blood in the left ventricle at the end of a full relaxation. That number is then divided by the volume of blood at the end of a full relaxation, and the result is multiplied by 100 to define the EF as a percentage.
- If your EF is less than 35 percent, talk to your doctor about whether you might benefit from an implantable cardioverter defibrillator.
- If your EF is greater than 50 percent, you are less likely to need an implantable defibrillator. An exception is hypertrophic cardiomyopathy, a condition in which the heart muscle is thickened and its contraction is very strong (hyperdynamic). The EF in this condition may be greater than 70 percent. If you have hypertrophic cardiomyopathy, you may be at risk for sudden death from ventricular arrhythmias, especially if your heart muscle is very thick or your family has a history of sudden death, ventricular tachycardia, or syncope (sudden loss of consciousness).

TABLE 5.2   *What does your ejection fraction (EF) mean?*

EF (%)	Severity of heart weakness
50 or greater	Normal
40 to 49	Mild heart weakness
30 to 39	Moderate heart weakness
Less than 30	Severe heart weakness

An EF less than 50 percent is abnormal. Depending on your symptoms and medical history, and whether you have ventricular tachycardia, if your EF is between 35 and 50, you might also benefit from an ICD. Discuss your EF number with your cardiologist, who may advise you to see an electrophysiologist (heart rhythm specialist) who can assist in the decision process.

Keep in mind that people with a seemingly normal EF can have a condition called *hypertrophic cardiomyopathy*. People with this condition have a thickened heart muscle with a very strong heart contraction (EF greater than 50 percent and possibly even greater than 70 percent). This condition may put a person at risk for sudden death from ventricular arrhythmias, especially if the heart muscle is very thick or if the patient has a family history of sudden death, ventricular tachycardia, or syncope (sudden loss of consciousness).

PART TWO

Heart Rhythm Abnormalities

CHAPTER 6

Slow Rhythms
Bradycardias

....

Any abnormality in heart rate and rhythm—whether it is too fast, too slow, "skips" a beat, races, or is irregular—is considered an arrhythmia. There are many different kinds of arrhythmias. A heart rate of fewer than 60 beats per minute may be called a slow rhythm, or bradycardia (*brady* means "slow"). A pause is a slowing of the heart rate and is evaluated by how long there is no electrical activity. Such a rhythm may not be clinically significant unless the person is experiencing symptoms such as fatigue, shortness of breath, light-headedness, dizziness, or loss of consciousness (also called *syncope*).

Slow rhythms are sometimes caused by medications. For example, beta blockers, calcium channel blockers, and digitalis might slow down the heart rate and cause bradycardia (table 6.1). Some antiarrhythmic drugs, such as sotalol and amiodarone, which have properties similar to beta blockers and calcium channel blockers, can also cause bradycardia.

These slow rhythms may also be caused by an underactive thyroid (hypothyroidism); an infection such as Lyme disease; or intrinsic disease of the heart's conduction system, caused by lack of blood

TABLE 6.1 *Medications that may cause bradycardia*

Beta blockers	Digitalis
Calcium channel blockers	Antiarrhythmic drugs such as sotalol and amiodarone

flow, long-standing hypertension, scarring, calcification, fibrosis, or some other condition. Bradycardia caused by hypothyroidism and Lyme disease may be treated with medications that address the underlying condition (thyroid replacement for hypothyroidism and antibiotics for Lyme disease). Occasionally the person's heart needs to be supplemented with temporary artificial pacing (stimulation) until the medications adequately treat the underlying problem.

Reversible causes of bradycardia, such as drug toxicity and electrolyte abnormalities, are listed in table 6.2. For common types of slow heart rhythms, see table 6.3.

One of the most common slow rhythms is sinus bradycardia, in which the SA node is sluggish in initiating electrical impulses to the heart. Second-degree heart block means that some of the impulses from the atria do not arrive at the ventricles. In Mobitz type I second-degree AV block, there is progressive delay in the AV node, and the doctor can recognize a clear pattern of grouped beating on an electrical recording of the heart rhythm called an electrocardiogram (ECG or EKG; see chapter 14). This condition may not be significant, especially if the patient has no symptoms. In Mobitz type II second-degree heart block, the loss of conduction of an atrial beat to the ventricle occurs suddenly, without any ECG pattern of delay (again, however, the doctor can recognize it). In third-degree heart block, also called *complete heart block*, none of the impulses from the atria conduct to the ventricles. Conduction disease in Mobitz type II second-degree heart block and third-degree heart block are usually at the level of the His bundle or lower. Finally, no heart contraction at all for a prolonged period is called *asystole,* regardless of what is causing it. The ECG is a simple noninvasive test used to record and identify various heart rhythm abnormalities (see chapter 14). An ECG strip of a sinus bradycardia in which the heart rate

TABLE 6.2 *Reversible causes of bradycardia*

Nonessential medications	Electrolyte abnormality
Lyme disease	Drug toxicity
Hypothyroidism	

TABLE 6.3 *Common types of slow heart rhythms*

Sinus bradycardia

Second-degree heart block, Mobitz type I (block typically occurs in the AV node)

Second-degree heart block, Mobitz type II (block typically occurs in the His bundle or below)

Third-degree heart block or complete heart block

Asystole

is fewer than 60 beats per minute is shown in figure 14.3 on page 61.

Significant bradycardia due to intrinsic conduction disease or essential medications, in which the heart rate is lower than 40 beats per minute or pauses are greater than 3 seconds, may require implantation of a permanent pacemaker if the patient has symptoms such as tiredness and fatigue, shortness of breath, light-headedness and dizziness, or loss of consciousness. Bradycardia occurring as the result of high-grade heart block (Mobitz type II second-degree AV block or third-degree AV block) may also require treatment with a permanent pacemaker, even in the absence of symptoms. If asystole is not due to a reversible cause, a permanent pacemaker may be required. If you have a slow rhythm and your doctor does not suggest that you get a pacemaker, ask your doctor whether you need one and find out why or why not. That way you are communicating about a treatment that you may need now, later, or never.

CHAPTER 7

Fast Rhythms

Tachycardias

....

Normal impulses originate in the SA node, which is located in the top part of the right atrial chamber. If the SA node fires at rates greater than 100 beats per minute, this is known as *tachycardia* (*tachy* means "fast"). At rest (when you are resting or being still), your heart rate should be no greater than 100 beats per minute, while during exercise, your heart rate may increase well above 100 beats per minute. An increase in heart rate during exertion is a normal response and is called *appropriate sinus tachycardia*. If you take your pulse while exercising, you will find that your heart rate is higher than it is at rest. If you take your pulse a few minutes after exercising, you will find that your heart rate has returned to a normal rate (though it might stay elevated for a while after exertion).

Some common types of fast heart rhythms are listed in Table 7.1. The first five tachycardias on the list are supraventricular tachycardias (occurring above the ventricles). Sinus tachycardia, probably the most common problem, originates in the SA node, is often benign, and does not require treatment. Rarely, this condition is considered *inappropriate sinus tachycardia*, especially when it is not due to a physiological condition or situation (such as an infection, low blood count, or anemia). Atrial fibrillation is a common type of arrhythmia in which the upper chamber moves very chaotically and rapidly. It is often referred to as an irregular rhythm. Atrial flutter is a more regular version of atrial fibrillation. Atrial tachycardia is often the result of a focus, or spot, within the atrium firing at a rapid

TABLE 7.1 *Common types of fast heart rhythms*

Sinus tachycardia (often benign)	Paroxysmal supraventricular
Atrial fibrillation	tachycardia (PSVT)
Atrial flutter	Ventricular tachycardia
Atrial tachycardia	Ventricular fibrillation

rate (but typically slower than atrial flutter or fibrillation). Paroxysmal supraventricular tachycardia (PSVT) often involves an extra connection (called an *accessory pathway*) within the heart, either in the AV node or outside it. This type of tachycardia has a very high cure rate with a procedure known as *catheter ablation*.

Ventricular tachycardia and ventricular fibrillation, in which the lower chambers of the heart beat very rapidly, are the leading causes of sudden cardiac arrest. If a person has ventricular tachycardia or fibrillation and becomes unconscious, his or her condition should be treated very quickly by defibrillation. People at risk for this condition should be considered for an implantable defibrillator.

The ECG tracing shown in figure 7.1 is of a normal heart rhythm, also known as *normal sinus rhythm*. Some people may experience fast heart rates at rest, which may be considered inappropriate sinus tachycardia. Some fast heart rhythms may originate in other locations throughout the heart. Depending on where the

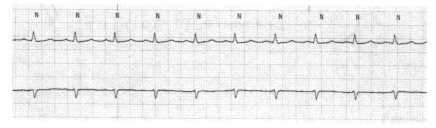

FIGURE 7.1. An electrical recording of the heart is called an electrocardiogram (ECG or EKG; see chapter 14 for more information). This ECG tracing shows a normal heart rhythm, also called normal sinus rhythm. The heart rate for normal sinus rhythm is between 60 and 100 beats per minute.

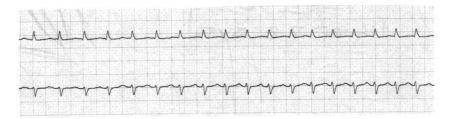

FIGURE 7.2.   An ECG tracing of an abnormal heart rhythm called supraventricular tachycardia, when the heart is beating at greater than 100 beats per minute. This patient's heart is beating regularly at 188 beats per minute. The precise type of supraventricular tachycardia may be difficult to discern with only one or two ECG leads.

impulses originate, these might be called *supraventricular tachycardias*, when they originate above the ventricles, or ventricular tachycardias, when their point of origin is in the ventricles.

An ECG strip of a supraventricular tachycardia, originating from the upper chambers of the heart, is shown in figure 7.2. The type of supraventricular tachycardia is either atrial fibrillation or atrial flutter (see chapters 9, 10, and 11) and is better defined if a more complete, twelve-lead ECG is performed. Signs and symptoms of fast heart rhythms include:

palpitations
dizziness
light-headedness
shortness of breath
loss of consciousness (syncope)

An abnormally fast rhythm can lead to a life-threatening situation. If you experience any of these symptoms, *contact your doctor or call 911.*

CHAPTER 8

Ventricular Tachycardia and Ventricular Fibrillation

....

Death from sudden cardiac arrest is usually caused by an arrhythmia. Most people who die from sudden cardiac arrest experience a fast heart rhythm from the lower chamber of the heart known as *ventricular tachycardia.* Many of them have heart disease as the result of coronary artery disease and have possibly had a previous heart attack. Others have a weakening or thickening of the heart muscle from some other cause, such as a failing heart structure (valve disease) or long-standing high blood pressure. Some people have a genetic condition (see chapter 35) in which ventricular arrhythmias occur even though the person has a structurally normal heart.

Ventricular tachycardia is a rapid rhythm from the lower chamber of the heart (see figure 8.1). Ventricular tachycardia typically originates in the left ventricle and less frequently in the right ventricle.

When the rhythm is less organized and the lower chamber of the heart is quivering instead of contracting and pumping, the rhythm is termed *ventricular fibrillation.* The most effective way to treat this abnormal rhythm is with a defibrillator. This device can deliver a shock to the patient to break the ventricular tachycardia or fibrillation and restore a normal heart rhythm. An external version of the defibrillator is commonly seen on TV and in movies, in which paddles are placed on the chest and a shock is delivered to stop the arrhythmia and restore a more normal rhythm. An implantable

FIGURE 8.1. Ventricular tachycardia, originating from the lower chamber of the heart (the ventricle). The arrows demonstrate the starting point of this rapid rhythm (in this figure, the ventricular tachycardia originates in the left ventricle). LA = left atrium, LV = left ventricle, RA = right atrium, RV = right ventricle. (See also color version.)

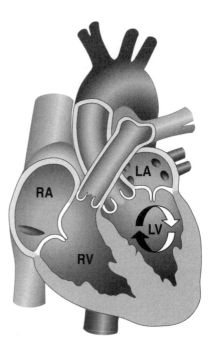

FIGURE 8.2. An implantable cardioverter defibrillator (ICD) pulse generator. This device is connected to at least one wire, which is typically inserted through a blood vessel into the heart. Your doctor may prescribe an ICD if you are at risk for sudden cardiac death. It helps to treat lethal arrhythmias such as ventricular tachycardia and ventricular fibrillation. Note that the specific type of ICD shown in this figure is a biventricular device (see chapter 28).

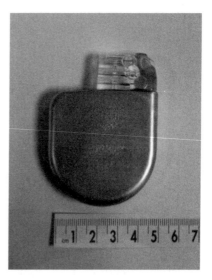

version, called an *implantable cardioverter defibrillator* (ICD), can perform the same task without delay and can improve survival in high-risk patients. An ICD generator is pictured in figure 8.2.

CHAPTER 9

Supraventricular Tachycardia

All the fast rhythms described in the following chapters may fall into a larger category of rhythms that generally occur from the atria (or the upper chambers) and are known as *supraventricular tachycardias*. Many of these rhythms can be treated with medications or cured by an intervention called a catheter ablation (see chapter 23).

One type of rhythm occurs when a person has an extra connection between the upper chamber (atrium) and the lower chamber (ventricle). When the extra connection falls within the AV node, the arrhythmia is called *AV node reentrant tachycardia*. The AV node normally has one pathway, but in this case two pathways are present (typically a fast one and a slow one). To treat this condition, catheter ablation can be highly effective at destroying the slow pathway of the AV node and leaving a fast pathway for normal conduction.

Another form of extra connection between the atria and ventricles but outside the AV node is called an accessory pathway. People experiencing symptoms of a fast rhythm (see chapter 7) who also have evidence of this pathway on their ECG have a condition known as Wolff-Parkinson-White syndrome. This disorder can lead to a rapid rhythm with the potential for loss of consciousness and even sudden cardiac arrest. Catheter ablation is very helpful at eliminating the extra pathway(s) and curing this disorder in a high percentage of patients.

Atrial fibrillation and atrial flutter, two common disorders, are examples of supraventricular tachycardias. They can lead to a nidus (a structure that looks and acts like a nest) for clot formation in the left atrium, which might increase a person's risk for a stroke. Anticoagulants (blood thinners) alone or with antiplatelet medications are often prescribed for such a condition, depending on the person's medical history. People older than 75 years, and people with congestive heart failure, diabetes, hypertension, or a prior stroke may also benefit from anticoagulant medications. A single episode of atrial fibrillation in a patient with a structurally normal heart and no other medical abnormalities might be treated with aspirin alone.

Typical atrial flutter can be easily cured by catheter ablation, but atrial fibrillation requires a more invasive ablative approach (see chapter 10). Other forms of supraventricular tachycardias, such as atrial tachycardias, are often the result of focal areas of atrial tissue firing at rapid rates. This rhythm can also be treated with catheter ablation and medications.

Atrial Fibrillation

One of the most common abnormal heart rhythms, atrial fibrillation, occurs when the upper chambers (atria) move very fast. This common rhythm occurs more often in older people than in young people and may be a result of long-standing high blood pressure or other heart disease. The quivering of the atria in atrial fibrillation is illustrated in figure 10.1.

A heart rate that is poorly controlled may stretch or weaken the heart muscle and cause shortness of breath, fatigue, light-headedness, and dizziness. Therefore, controlling the rate with medications is important. Another effect of atrial fibrillation is an increased risk of stroke or mini-stroke (especially in people with congestive heart failure, high blood pressure, diabetes, or advanced age).

Risk factors for atrial fibrillation are listed in table 10.1. People who have these risk factors are more likely to develop the condition. Early treatment of atrial fibrillation and aggressive treatment of these risk factors may help to prevent atrial fibrosis (scarring), which may result in persistent atrial fibrillation. At the Atrial Fibrillation Summit of the 2009 Heart Rhythm Scientific Sessions, there was talk about using aggressive treatment with angiotensin-converting enzyme inhibitors (also called ACE inhibitors) and statins (medications used to treat high cholesterol) to prevent progression to persistent atrial fibrillation. Further research is necessary to determine whether this is the proper approach to treatment, but in the meantime, it may be reasonable to proceed with these therapies,

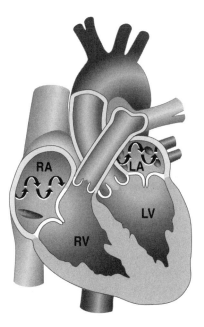

FIGURE 10.1. Atrial fibrillation is a fast rhythm that originates in the upper chambers of the heart, or atria. In many cases, atrial fibrillation may be caused by triggers that start from the pulmonary veins and then proceed into the left atrium. Catheter ablation in which the pulmonary veins are isolated from the left atrium can help treat some forms of atrial fibrillation. The arrows depict the fibrillation of the top chambers. LA = left atrium, LV = left ventricle, RA = right atrium, RV = right ventricle. (See also color version.)

TABLE 10.1   *Risk factors for atrial fibrillation*

High blood pressure (hypertension)	Open heart surgery
Diabetes	Chronic obstructive lung disease
Congestive heart failure	Sleep apnea
Coronary artery disease	Obesity
Myocardial infarction	Age (more common as we get
Thyroid disease	older)

especially if the person has lipid disorders (such as high cholesterol) and high blood pressure or congestive heart failure.

For a summary of important facts about atrial fibrillation, see table 10.2. In this table, "atrial fibrillation begets atrial fibrillation" means that the longer you are in atrial fibrillation, the longer you are likely to stay in atrial fibrillation. It has been demonstrated that long-standing atrial fibrillation can lead to scarring of the atrial heart muscle tissue. It may be possible to prevent or slow down this scarring process with early and aggressive treatment of atrial fibrillation and its risk factors (as noted above, treatment may include statins and ACE inhibitors).

Blood thinners (anticoagulants) are helpful in preventing stroke, especially if the person has risk factors for stroke. The memory device CHADS2 has been used to help identify these risk factors: Congestive heart failure, Hypertension, Age, Diabetes, Stroke (2 times more important than the other risks).

Medications are typically first-line treatment for atrial fibrillation. If patients are symptomatic from their fibrillation, heart rhythm drugs (antiarrhythmic drugs) may be used to help suppress this rhythm, along with anticoagulation if indicated. When patients remain symptomatic and fail to respond to antiarrhythmic medications, their doctor may consider catheter ablation (see chapter 23) the best treatment.

Atrial fibrillation ablation is an invasive transseptal procedure in which catheters are placed from the right side of the heart through the septum (the tissue that separates the atria) to the left side. Ablation is typically performed in the left atrium around the outside of pulmonary vein openings (the veins that attach to the left atrium) to prevent electrical triggers, which occur within the veins, from escaping into the left atrium and triggering atrial fibrillation. In essence, once these veins become isolated, the electrical triggers within the veins are unable to travel into the atrium, and atrial fibrillation cannot occur through this route. This form of atrial fibrillation ablation is a pulmonary vein isolation (PVI) procedure.

In addition, the doctor may ablate other areas in the left atrium

TABLE 10.2   *Atrial fibrillation facts*

- Atrial fibrillation is a very common heart rhythm problem.
- It is known as an "irregular rhythm."
- The chance of developing atrial fibrillation increases with age; according to recent statistics from the American Heart Association, atrial fibrillation may be found in 3 to 5 percent of people over the age of 65 (see table 10.1 for other atrial fibrillation risk factors).
- Atrial fibrillation begets atrial fibrillation (i.e., the longer you are in atrial fibrillation, the longer you stay in atrial fibrillation).
- Early treatment may help slow down the progression to persistent atrial fibrillation.
- Blood thinners (anticoagulants) are recommended in patients with congestive heart failure, hypertension, age greater than 75 years, diabetes, or history of stroke.
- First-line treatment is medication, including antiarrhythmic drugs.
- If antiarrhythmic drug therapy fails, catheter ablation should be considered.
- Inciting causes should also be treated: excess alcohol consumption, ischemia, hypertension, stimulant use, and thyroid disorders.

by creating lines, or ablating areas of continuous electrical activity. Ablation may be necessary in the right atrium as well. This procedure is one of the most invasive that electrophysiologists perform. Unfortunately, more than one procedure is often necessary to completely suppress the atrial fibrillation.

The best outcomes occur in patients who have relatively normal hearts and who go in and out of atrial fibrillation on their own (called *paroxysmal atrial fibrillation*). People who are elderly or have significantly abnormal heart structures and who have been in atrial fibrillation for a long time (also called *persistent*, or *chronic*, atrial fibrillation) are less likely to be cured by an ablation than people with paroxysmal atrial fibrillation. Complications from this procedure include bleeding, blood clots, vascular damage, damage to heart structures, perforation of the heart or blood vessels, heart attack, stroke, occlusion of the pulmonary vein or veins (causing shortness of breath), development of a connection between the atrium and the esophagus, and death.

Occasionally, surgery can provide a useful adjunctive approach to treating atrial fibrillation, especially if it can be done while another heart surgery, such as mitral valve repair or replacement, is being performed. One such procedure is called the *maze procedure*, in which a "maze" is created within the left atrium to prevent the perpetuation of atrial fibrillation. Surgical procedures, even minimally invasive surgical procedures, usually have significant risks compared with catheter-based electrophysiology procedures such as catheter ablation.

The success rate for all these procedures continues to improve with advances in understanding of the disorder, newer techniques, and additional clinical experience. Your physician should be willing to fully discuss the risks and treatment options with you. It is worth emphasizing that the use of catheter ablation should be limited to symptomatic patients who have failed to improve with, or who cannot tolerate, heart rhythm (antiarrhythmic) medications.

A simpler, less invasive procedure called an *AV junction ablation* (or AVJ ablation) can be performed in people whose heart rates fail to be controlled despite multiple medications (typically three or more drugs). By ablating the AV node or junction, it is possible to prevent the electrical signals from the upper chambers (atria) from conducting to the lower chambers (ventricles). After AVJ ablation, the person requires a permanent pacemaker to maintain an adequate heart rate and regularize the rhythm. This procedure is much simpler to perform than atrial fibrillation ablation and may be useful in elderly people and in those with multiple medical problems who may not be good candidates for the atrial fibrillation ablation procedure. People who receive an AVJ ablation and pacemaker should be aware, however, that they will likely become dependent on the pacemaker to provide every beat to the heart. Also, the AVJ ablation does not cure atrial fibrillation, which means that these patients will still have to take anticoagulants. In contrast, patients may be cured by the more invasive and more complicated atrial fibrillation ablation and may be able to discontinue anticoagulants after prolonged monitoring and conclusive evidence of cure.

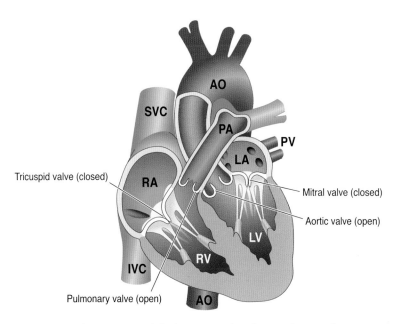

FIGURE 1.1.   The structure of the heart—its chambers, valves, and great vessels. AO = aorta, IVC = inferior vena cava, LA = left atrium, LV = left ventricle, PA = pulmonary artery, PV = pulmonary veins, RA = right atrium, RV = right ventricle, SVC = superior vena cava.

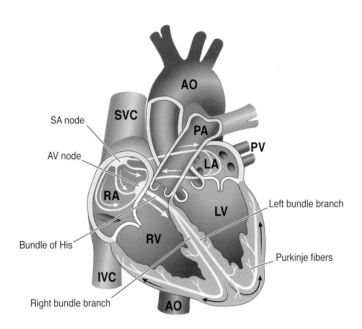

FIGURE 1.2. The conduction system of the heart. The arrows show the electrical impulses, which begin in the sinus, or sinoatrial, node and travel through the atria to the atrioventricular node. After a slight delay there, these impulses are conducted through the His bundle and through the right and left bundle branches to specialized Purkinje fibers, which carry the impulses into the ventricles. AO = aorta, AV node = atrioventricular node, IVC = inferior vena cava, LA = left atrium, LV = left ventricle, PA = pulmonary artery, PV = pulmonary veins, RA = right atrium, RV = right ventricle, SA node = sinus node, SVC = superior vena cava.

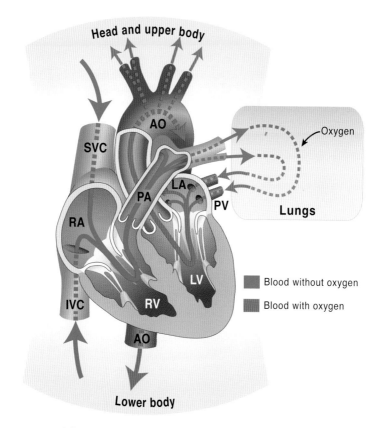

FIGURE 1.3. The sequence of circulation. The blue arrows show blood deprived of oxygen (deoxygenated blood) returning to the right side of the heart. The blood is then pumped to the lungs to receive oxygen. Oxygenated blood, indicated by red arrows, returns to the heart via the pulmonary veins and is then pumped from the left side of the heart to the rest of the body. AO = aorta, IVC = inferior vena cava, LA = left atrium, LV = left ventricle, PA = pulmonary artery, PV = pulmonary veins, RA = right atrium, RV = right ventricle, SVC = superior vena cava.

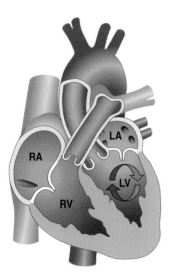

FIGURE 8.1. Ventricular tachycardia, originating from the lower chamber of the heart (the ventricle). The red arrows demonstrate the starting point of this rapid rhythm (in this figure, the ventricular tachycardia originates in the left ventricle). LA = left atrium, LV = left ventricle, RA = right atrium, RV = right ventricle.

FIGURE 10.1. Atrial fibrillation is a fast rhythm that originates in the upper chambers of the heart, or atria. In many cases, atrial fibrillation may be caused by triggers that start from the pulmonary veins and then proceed into the left atrium. Catheter ablation in which the pulmonary veins are isolated from the left atrium can help treat some forms of atrial fibrillation. The arrows depict the fibrillation of the top chambers. LA = left atrium, LV = left ventricle, RA = right atrium, RV = right ventricle.

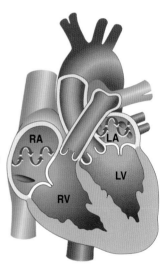

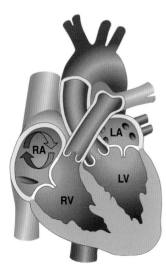

FIGURE 11.1. Atrial flutter is a rapid abnormal heart rhythm that originates from the upper chambers (atria). This figure illustrates typical atrial flutter, which originates in the right atrium. The arrows depict a larger, more organized rhythm than found with atrial fibrillation (see figure 10.1). LA = left atrium, LV = left ventricle, RA = right atrium, RV = right ventricle.

CHAPTER 11

Atrial Flutter

....

Atrial flutter is similar to atrial fibrillation in that the atrium beats very rapidly. However, the atrial rhythm usually has a more organized pattern than that of atrial fibrillation. Atrial flutter arising from the right atrium of the heart is depicted in figure 11.1. An ECG tracing of atrial flutter (figure 11.2) demonstrates jagged, or sawtooth, waves (regularized atrial activity, or P waves) between the ventricular events (QRS complexes; see chapter 14).

The electrical waves causing atrial flutter move in a circular rhythm through a funnel-like structure called the *isthmus*. If a line is drawn by catheter ablation across this critical area, the rhythm can easily be cured (see chapter 23 for a thorough discussion of catheter ablation). This circumstance makes ablation of this condition comparatively simple. In typical atrial flutter, which occurs in the right atrium, there is no need to perform a more risky transseptal puncture to get to the left side of the heart (as is true for atrial fibrillation ablation).

Catheter ablation of typical atrial flutter can be performed by placing a catheter across the tricuspid valve and ablating down to the inferior vena cava. The clinician's experience often dictates how long this procedure will take and how effective it will be.

Alternatively, medications can be used to treat and control this arrhythmia. People who require cardioversion (breaking of the rhythm) and people with risk factors for stroke (see chapter 10) may need to take anticoagulants (blood thinners). Some key facts about atrial flutter are presented in table 11.1.

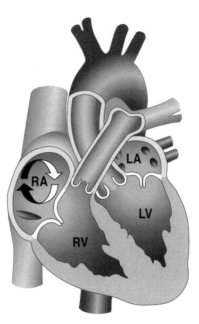

FIGURE 11.1. Atrial flutter is a rapid abnormal heart rhythm that originates from the upper chambers (atria). This figure illustrates typical atrial flutter, which originates in the right atrium. The arrows depict a larger, more organized rhythm than found with atrial fibrillation (see figure 10.1). LA = left atrium, LV = left ventricle, RA = right atrium, RV = right ventricle. (See also color version.)

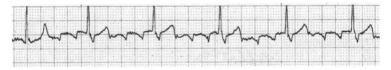

FIGURE 11.2. Atrial flutter is similar to atrial fibrillation; however, the atrial rhythm is more regular and organized. This ECG strip shows rapid, regular, jagged (or sawtooth) waves coming from the atrium before each ventricular event.

TABLE 11.1 *Atrial flutter facts*

- Atrial flutter is more organized than atrial fibrillation.
- Atrial flutter should be treated like atrial fibrillation with respect to medications, including blood thinners (anticoagulants).
- Atrial flutter is much easier to cure with catheter ablation than atrial fibrillation is. Catheter ablation can be considered a first-line therapy for symptomatic atrial flutter.
- Catheter ablation success rates for the typical forms of atrial flutter are higher than those achieved with atrial fibrillation.

PART THREE

Sudden Cardiac Arrest

CHAPTER 12

Sudden Cardiac Arrest

Sudden cardiac arrest is the condition in which a patient collapses suddenly due to a heart rhythm abnormality. In the United States, sudden cardiac arrest takes a life every two minutes — nearly 1,000 individuals each day. Unfortunately, this all-too-common problem may account for more deaths than cancer and acquired immunodeficiency syndrome (AIDS) combined.

Heart rhythm problems that may cause sudden cardiac arrest are listed in table 12.1. The event is most often associated with rapid rhythms from the lower chamber, called ventricular tachycardia or ventricular fibrillation. The heart rhythm problems that cause sudden cardiac arrest most often affect people who have heart disease (an abnormal heart) caused by a heart attack, blockages of the coronary arteries, a weak heart muscle, thick heart muscles, or other problems.

The best treatment for sudden cardiac arrest from ventricular tachycardia or ventricular fibrillation is rapid defibrillation (electrical shock therapy). Defibrillation is a procedure in which electrical energy (direct current energy) is delivered to terminate the tachycardia or fibrillation and restore a normal rhythm. When the cause of the ventricular tachycardia or fibrillation cannot be reversed, an implantable cardioverter defibrillator (ICD) is the best treatment.

Sudden cardiac arrest is also caused (though less often) by supraventricular tachycardia (rhythm problems from the upper chambers of the heart) and slow heart rhythms (bradycardias), as a result

TABLE 12.1   *Heart rhythm causes of sudden cardiac arrest*

Fast heart rhythms (tachycardias)	Slow heart rhythms (bradycardias)

Ventricular tachycardia
Ventricular fibrillation
Supraventricular tachycardia
  (less frequent)
	Complete or high-grade heart
	  block
	Asystole

of either a severe blockage in the electrical wiring system between the upper and lower heart chambers, or the cessation of electrical impulses altogether (a condition called asystole). These two types of bradycardias are typically treated with an implantable device called a *permanent pacemaker*, which delivers electrical impulses to the heart (see chapter 26).

The reversible causes of sudden cardiac arrest are listed in table 12.2. Reversible causes include drug toxicity, electrolyte abnormalities, or a blocked coronary artery depriving the heart of oxygen from its blood supply. These reversible causes can be treated by discontinuing the drug, treating the electrolyte abnormality, or opening or bypassing the blocked coronary artery. Treating these causes of sudden cardiac arrest may not necessarily include an ICD, especially if the treatments just mentioned successfully reverse the problem.

Coronary artery disease develops as the result of fat and calcium deposits forming plaques within the coronary arteries, a process called *atherosclerosis*. The link between atherosclerosis and sudden cardiac arrest is described in table 12.3. The plaques that build up can rupture within the artery, blocking the heart muscle's supply of blood and oxygen. When blood and oxygen are cut off, ventricular tachycardia or ventricular fibrillation may result. After the patient is successfully resuscitated and defibrillated, the doctor may find changes in the ECG suggesting that the patient has had an acute myocardial infarction or has ischemia. A test called a *coronary angiogram* can show the location of this newly blocked coronary artery. A percutaneous coronary intervention (PCI), such as an angioplasty, may be performed to open the blockage.

TABLE 12.2   *Reversible causes of sudden cardiac arrest*

Cause	Treatment
Drug toxicity	Remove toxic drug
Electrolyte abnormalities	Correct electrolyte abnormality
Blocked coronary artery	Remove blockage (stent) or bypass blockage (surgery)

Note: These conditions don't necessarily require an ICD.

TABLE 12.3   *The link between atherosclerosis and sudden cardiac arrest*

Atherosclerosis: buildup of calcium and fatty deposits in the arterial walls.

Consequences: coronary artery disease (CAD), which may manifest itself as chest pain (angina), heart attack, arrhythmias, or sudden cardiac arrest. When blood supply to the brain and limbs is impaired, atherosclerosis can cause mini-strokes, strokes, and peripheral arterial disease.

Links to sudden cardiac arrest:
- Two-thirds of Americans (approximately 2 million) have some plaque buildup (CAD) by age 35.
- Each year approximately 800,000 Americans have their first heart attack, and 500,000 Americans will have a recurring attack (according to the American Heart Association).
- CAD with a prior heart attack is a leading risk factor for sudden cardiac arrest.
- Sudden cardiac arrest kills nearly 300,000 Americans each year.

Source: Derived from the Sudden Cardiac Arrest Association, "Fact Sheet: Atherosclerosis and SCA."

An angioplasty involves placing a balloon catheter into a coronary artery to open the blood vessel. A stent (an expandable piece of metal similar to the spring inside a pen) may or may not be inserted across the opened blockage to keep the coronary artery open. Stents may be made of bare metal or may be coated with drugs, depending on what the physician believes is best for the patient. Coronary artery bypass surgery may be required when the coronary artery disease is extensive or too dangerous to be treated by a PCI.

Treatment following coronary artery revascularization procedures such as a stent or bypass surgery includes preventive measures such as diet, lifestyle changes, and medications to stall progression of coronary artery disease and avoid reocclusion of the stent (see chapter 36). An ICD may be required if revascularization is not complete or if a heart attack damaged a significant amount of the heart muscle (especially if this damage persists beyond 90 days). An ICD may not be required in patients who suffered sudden cardiac arrest due to a blocked coronary artery, especially if the heart function is not impaired and the blockage is corrected. My recommendation, however, is that the patient's household be trained in cardiopulmonary resuscitation (CPR) and consider purchasing an automatic external defibrillator (AED) in case of emergency.

The limited availability of AEDs throughout the community is a problem. Outside the hospital setting, most people who experience sudden cardiac arrest will die before emergency help arrives. This situation has raised awareness in communities and has led to grassroots efforts to provide cities, suburbs, and rural areas with AEDs. Find out where in your local community AEDs are located. They are now found in many public places, such as airports, sports arenas, and community sports playing fields.

Patients who are at risk for heart disease in general are also at risk for heart rhythm problems, including ventricular tachycardia and ventricular fibrillation (and sudden cardiac arrest). There are a few things you should know if you or a loved one is at risk for sudden cardiac arrest (table 12.4). Anyone at risk must work with his or her doctor(s) to prevent and treat risk factors. Steps include stopping smoking, treating high blood pressure and high cholesterol, treating diabetes, eating healthfully, and losing weight. Patients and their friends and family members should learn resuscitation methods such as CPR and proper use of an AED. In addition, people at risk for heart disease should know how to get help, and they or their loved ones should call 911 if they have symptoms of sudden cardiac arrest:

chest pain
pressure or discomfort in the chest

very rapid heart palpitations
significant light-headedness or dizziness
loss of consciousness

People at risk for sudden cardiac arrest should know their ejection fraction (EF; see chapter 5). If their EF is reduced (35 percent or lower), they should talk to their doctor about whether they need an ICD.

If you or a family member is at risk for sudden cardiac arrest, all family members should be trained in CPR. Read the patient's story at the end of this chapter to appreciate why learning CPR is so important. Classes are available through the American Heart Association (AHA), the American Red Cross, and many local hospitals. For more information, contact AHA toll-free at 800-242-8721 or visit www.heart.org.

Support groups have been established for anyone who wants to and can attend. These groups provide educational and emotional support for people affected by sudden cardiac arrest (see chapter 40). In addition, the Sudden Cardiac Arrest Association hosts a Web site with an extensive library of resources, including a patient discussion forum. You can contact this group at www.suddencardiac arrest.org or toll free at 866-972-7222.

One patient's story begins on the next page.

TABLE 12.4 *Preventing and treating sudden cardiac arrest*

- Know your risk factors for heart disease (see table 36.2). These include family history, age, high blood pressure, high cholesterol, diabetes, obesity, smoking, poor diet, and sedentary lifestyle.
- Know how to treat risk factors (see table 36.2): Take care of your health through diet, exercise, stress reduction, and medications (as prescribed by your doctor).
- Know your EF (ejection fraction). If your EF is 35 percent or less, ask your doctor if you can benefit from an ICD.
- Know how to get help in an emergency: call 911.
- Know how to perform CPR (see chapter 37).
- Know how to use an automatic external defibrillator (see chapter 38).

I was fortunate, at age 56, to be active enough to play in a 40 and over softball league. In the ten years that I had been playing in the league, not one single player ever sustained any on-the-field injury more serious than a pulled muscle, although that happened quite frequently.

One evening while playing at Oceanside High School, the last thing I remember is taking my position at third base in the fourth inning and talking with a friend of mine on the other team. I have since been told that I returned to the dugout, sat down, and keeled over. Fortunately, one of my friends called 911 and another friend, who had CPR training but had never had to use it on a real person, started to bang away at my chest. It turns out that they had followed the recommended guidelines by immediately calling 911 and by starting CPR. My friend who had started the CPR has since told me that he really didn't know what he was doing, but he had been taught that doing something was better than doing nothing.

The high school was conducting a review course that evening, and just as my incident occurred, the students were being let out of the school. Two of them saw what had happened and they ran to their mothers, who immediately came to my rescue. One of them was a nurse, and the other was a former EMT worker. I have come to think of them as angels who were sent by God to save me. I will be forever grateful to them. The police arrived within three minutes, and they successfully defibrillated me. I had several burn marks to prove that.

The next thing I remember is being in some confined space and someone whom I had never met telling me that I was a lucky guy. I had a very hard time comprehending what was happening to me, but I knew that I was still alive. My initial thoughts were to ask the people around me to tell my wife that I was OK, and from that point on, my foremost thoughts have been for her and not for myself. I next recall being wheeled into the emergency room and seeing my wife and children and my brother and his family.

I had visited numerous friends and family members in the hospital over the years, and it was very unusual and uncomfortable to be the one in the hospital bed. I had always been the one bringing the flowers. I thought back a few years, when I had seen my father in a cardiac care unit in Florida after he had undergone a mitral valve replacement, and I recalled how sorry I had felt for him and how helpless he had looked. I felt just as helpless now. I had always been the rock of my family, their provider and protector, and here I was, the subject of their fear and concern. I had to first reassure them, and then myself, that I would be fine and that we'd get through this together.

The next few days were a blur. After meeting some wonderful nurses that night, I met my doctor, a fine, warm, and caring cardiologist who discussed my medical care with me as a new cardiac patient. I could not believe that he was actually talking to me about the necessity of undergoing a cardiac catheterization the next morning to determine the cause of my cardiac arrest. As he explained to me that he might need to place stents in me or, if my case was more serious, that I might need cardiac bypass surgery, it seemed as if he was talking about someone else. I was still having trouble believing that he was talking about me.

The procedure itself went quickly, and I remember the doctor's reassuring words. He had found two major blockages in the left anterior descending artery, which he had been able to treat with stents. I would not need bypass grafts, and I had not sustained any heart damage. He was the first of hundreds of people to tell me how lucky I was. I have since learned that a blockage in the left anterior descending artery is called "the widowmaker" and that sudden cardiac arrest victims have a 93 percent fatality rate. I started to struggle with the concept of why this had happened to me and why I had been saved.

The days and months following my cardiac arrest have been filled with thoughts about what happened and about what almost happened. Although I have come to understand that I would be fine physically, I initially felt older and less capable. I began to wonder why this happened to me and not to the thousands of other people who, I suddenly noticed, were terribly overweight and were eating things that I never would have eaten even before my event. I felt as if my world had been turned upside down, and I realized that the psychological effects on me could be greater than the physical effects.

I have come to learn much more about coronary artery disease than I ever thought I would. Before this incident, unfortunately, I took my health for granted. After working with several doctors, nurses, and nutritionists, I now understand that there are several risk factors everyone can control or modify. I also understand why most people don't pay much attention to this. They just don't give any thought to the idea that it could happen to them. Unfortunately, it took my incident for me to understand the importance of taking steps to become healthier in general.

PART FOUR

Syncope

CHAPTER 13

Syncope

....

Loss of consciousness—passing out or fainting—is called *syncope*. While syncope is often dismissed or self-diagnosed as "nothing to worry about," you should report any incident to your doctor. Repeated incidents of syncope should prompt you to see your doctor in an office visit. Fainting is one of the most common reasons people are brought to the emergency room or admitted to the hospital. The work-up for these patients (as with any heart rhythm patient) begins with a history, a physical examination, and an ECG performed by the medical team. If the history fails to identify any signs of a heart problem or any clinical clues that would lead to a specific diagnosis, a tilt table test may be useful (this is a noninvasive test in which the patient, on a table, is stood nearly erect and the heart rate and blood pressure are monitored; see chapter 22). If, on the other hand, the initial work-up identifies a heart rhythm–related risk factor or abnormality, the doctor will probably consider doing an electrophysiology study (an invasive test of the patient's heart rhythm and heart wiring system).

Common causes of syncope are listed in table 13.1. One is a condition called *neurocardiogenic*, or *vasovagal*, *syncope*, which may be triggered by standing for a long time. Under this circumstance, the body may release a hormone called *adrenaline*, which triggers the nervous system to respond. Sometimes this response is an overactivation of the vagus nerve (a nerve that originates in the brain and affects many structures, including the heart), which may

TABLE 13.1   *Causes of syncope*

Neurocardiogenic syncope or vasovagal syncope	Valve problems (aortic stenosis or mitral stenosis)
Dehydration	Seizure disorder or stroke
Heart rhythm problems	

cause the heart rate to slow and blood pressure to drop. The result of these physiological changes is a feeling of dizziness, and sometimes people pass out.

Dehydration is another cause of syncope. In this case, the body is deprived of fluid and nutrients, and the person can become symptomatic when changing position, such as going from lying down (supine) to sitting or standing. Less frequently, the cause of syncope is neurological, such as a stroke or a seizure.

Heart rhythm problems as well as heart valve disease, such as aortic or mitral stenosis, can cause syncope. People with these cardiac causes of syncope have the worst prognosis if the causes are not treated. Importantly, once diagnosed, many heart-related causes of syncope can be effectively treated with medications, catheter ablation, heart surgery, or an implantable device. Your doctor may prescribe a tilt table test to identify what is causing your syncope. If the cause of a person's syncope is thought to be cardiac related, and potentially heart rhythm related, an electrophysiology study will probably be considered. This test is useful for determining whether the patient has serious arrhythmias or conduction disease, and it can help guide effective treatment.

A thorough medical work-up may be helpful in identifying your problem and resolving the condition. If a complete work-up fails to uncover the cause of syncope, then an external or implantable cardiac monitor may be useful in elucidating a heart rhythm problem that may be causing the syncope. (Chapter 16 describes implantable cardiac monitors.) An implantable cardiac monitor can be helpful in finding the cause of infrequent syncope. In many people, slow heart rhythm problems (bradycardias) are uncovered and a pacemaker is then recommended.

TABLE 13.2   *Syncope facts*

- Syncope is one of the most common reasons a person visits the emergency room.
- Syncope from heart problems is often more serious (there is a higher chance of dying) than syncope from non-heart-related problems if the heart problems are not successfully treated.
- Heart-related syncope is often readily treatable.
- A tilt table test can be used to assess syncope, especially if the history, physical exam, and ECG fail to elucidate any significant cardiac findings.
- An electrophysiology study (invasive heart rhythm test) is useful, especially when heart rhythm–related abnormalities are discovered in the history, physical exam, or ECG.
- External or implantable cardiac monitors are often helpful in finding a heart rhythm problem related to syncope.
- Extensive neurological evaluations may not be necessary and should not be routine for each syncope episode, but they may be performed on a case-by-case basis.

For a summary of facts about syncope, see table 13.2. The American Heart Association Web site has additional information. See www.heart.org.

PART FIVE

The Tests

....

Board-certified cardiologists and electrophysiologists use the diagnostic and imaging tests and procedures described in chapters 14 to 22 to assess and identify heart rhythm problems and related conditions. Not every test is appropriate for every patient.

CHAPTER 14

Electrocardiogram (ECG or EKG)

An ECG is a simple, painless, noninvasive test that can be performed in virtually any clinic, doctor's office, or medical facility. Small electrodes are attached to the chest, arms, and legs, and then an image of the electrical signal as it is portrayed on the surface of your heart is printed on paper that runs through the recording device. The ECG can show changes that suggest a blocked coronary artery or a heart rhythm abnormality. For a summary of ECG facts, see table 14.1.

A typical twelve-lead ECG for a heart in which the upper and lower chambers beat in a normal sequence is shown in figure 14.1. A normal rhythm is called *normal sinus rhythm* (since it originates in the sinus node), and a normal heart rate is between 60 and 100 beats per minute.

From an ECG, it is possible to determine whether your rhythm is normal or abnormal. Abnormal rhythms include slow rhythms (bradycardias), fast rhythms (tachycardias), and heart block (in

TABLE 14.1 *ECG facts*

- An ECG is a simple, noninvasive test.
- Ask your physician for a copy of the paper tracing from your ECG and place it in your personal records. It is useful to have a copy available in case of an emergency or if you change or add physicians.
- Your ECG can show changes that could suggest a blocked coronary artery or a heart rhythm abnormality.

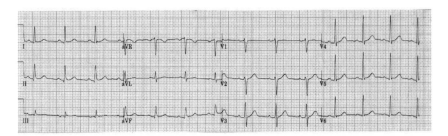

FIGURE 14.1. Standard twelve-lead electrocardiogram (ECG or EKG) showing a reading from a normal heart. A twelve-lead ECG is a baseline assessment of your heart. From this, your doctor can determine heart rhythm abnormalities. Your doctor may compare a previous twelve-lead ECG with your current ECG to see if there have been any significant changes.

which impulses from the atria fail to conduct to the ventricles). In addition, the ECG can show the effects of electrolytes (normal or abnormal blood chemistry) and medications on the heart.

A single ECG signal is depicted in figure 14.2. This figure shows the normal sequence of electrical activity of the heart recorded from the surface ECG. The electrical signal may be broken into different

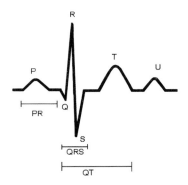

FIGURE 14.2. A single ECG recording of a heartbeat. This figure shows the normal electrical sequence of the heart. The electrical signal may be broken into different waves. The P wave represents atrial electrical activity; the QRS complex represents ventricular electrical activity; and the QT interval (from the beginning of the Q wave to the end of the T wave) represents the ventricles returning to a resting state.

waves. The medical terms P, QRS, T, and U are used to describe waves when referring to the ECG. The P wave represents atrial electrical activity; the QRS complex represents ventricular electrical activity; and the QT interval (from the beginning of the Q wave to the end of the T wave) represents the ventricles returning to a resting state, or repolarization, while the U wave represents relaxation of the Purkinje fibers of the conduction system.

A slower than normal rhythm (sinus bradycardia), in which the heart rate is below 60 beats per minute, is demonstrated in figure 14.3. If the rhythm *exceeded* 100 beats per minute, a sinus tachycardia would be present. In atrial fibrillation (figure 14.4), there are no discrete P waves present, but chaotic atrial activity can be seen between the QRS complexes. The atria are quivering and fail to efficiently pump the blood into the ventricles. An example of atrial flutter on an ECG, which can be identified by sawtooth P waves, is shown in chapter 11 (see figure 11.2).

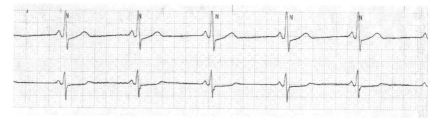

FIGURE 14.3. An ECG tracing demonstrating sinus bradycardia (slow heart rhythm) in which the heart is beating at approximately 46 beats per minute (normal is 60 to 100 beats per minute).

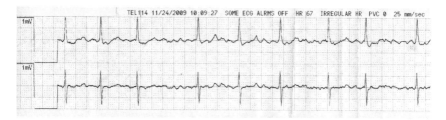

FIGURE 14.4. An ECG tracing demonstrating atrial fibrillation, a rapid atrial rhythm in which the P waves are irregular and chaotic.

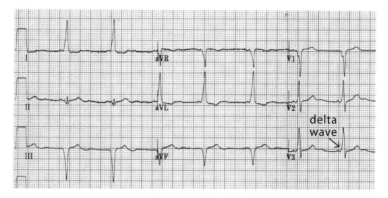

FIGURE 14.5. Part of a twelve-lead ECG of a patient with Wolff-Parkinson-White (WPW) syndrome. Note fusion from the end of the P wave to the QRS complex. This is called a delta wave, and it is highlighted by the arrow. Patients with WPW syndrome may be at risk for sudden cardiac arrest and may benefit from catheter ablation.

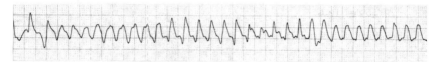

FIGURE 14.6. An ECG tracing of ventricular tachycardia. This is considered a life-threatening arrhythmia and requires prompt medical attention. If the condition is not due to a reversible cause, an ICD should be considered.

Wolff-Parkinson-White (WPW) syndrome is a condition in which there is an extra connection between the atrium and ventricle (accessory pathway). People with WPW have supraventricular tachycardia plus a characteristic baseline ECG in which a delta wave is present (fusion of the P wave and the QRS complex; figure 14.5).

An example of ventricular tachycardia is shown in figure 14.6. These impulses are originating in the ventricles and are firing at a rapid rate. The QRS complexes of ventricular tachycardia are typically wider than the normal baseline QRS complexes. If it does not resolve spontaneously, ventricular tachycardia usually requires defibrillation.

CHAPTER 15

Stress Test and Related Procedures

....

To identify whether your heart is performing normally, your doctor may order a stress test. It is considered a functional test because it determines how well your heart functions under stress. While you exercise, your heart must pump more blood because your body requires more oxygen. A doctor recommends a stress test to patients when he or she is diagnosing or ruling out coronary artery disease or checking the effectiveness of a previously performed PCI procedure (such as angioplasty and stenting). This test is also useful in predicting a person's risk of a heart attack. For people with a normal ECG who have been sedentary prior to beginning an exercise program, the stress test can evaluate their fitness for exercise. In addition, this test may be useful in determining a patient's fitness before he or she has major surgery.

In a stress test, you exercise on a treadmill while the ECG is monitored. Your walking or running speed is progressively increased along with the grade (or slope) as the doctor continuously analyzes your blood pressure as well as the ECG. Changes in the ECG recording and the development of arrhythmias during exercise-induced stress may indicate the presence of coronary artery disease.

Your doctor may also perform a nuclear stress test in which a nuclear agent (radioisotope) is injected into your vein and images of your heart are acquired to identify whether areas in the heart muscle are receiving enough blood. This study can also help determine if blockages are present. This test might be more useful in people with an abnormal ECG, a prior heart condition or heart-related risk factors, or body that is unusual or large. In addition to a regular nuclear stress test, certain drugs such as adenosine and dobutamine may be administered to help facilitate the test, especially if the patient cannot walk or run for any length of time. A stress test may be followed by an echocardiogram to help demonstrate whether the heart muscle itself functions appropriately under stress.

The most definitive test (although somewhat invasive) is a cardiac catheterization, also known as a coronary angiogram (see chapter 19). During this procedure, a tube (catheter) is inserted into the groin, and a catheter is inserted into the arteries that lead to the heart. Contrast dye is injected, and imaging may be performed through cinefluoroscopy (a type of radiation) to help diagnose a blockage. Discrete blockages can be effectively treated with a stent, and more extensive disease can be treated by coronary artery bypass surgery.

A review of some stress test facts is presented in table 15.1. Information for patients preparing for cardiac procedures is detailed in table 15.2. For all stress tests (including the tilt table test) and for all invasive procedures, the patient must have nothing by mouth (also called NPO) for at least 6 hours prior to the procedure. In addition, the doctor may ask the patient to stop taking blood thinners, such as warfarin (Coumadin), and antiplatelet medications,

TABLE 15.1 *Stress test facts*

- Stress tests are useful for diagnosing blockages and predicting heart attacks.
- They can reveal rhythm problems by bringing on symptoms.
- They are not as definitive as a cardiac catheterization, which shows pictures of the coronary arteries (the vessels that supply the heart with oxygenated blood).
- Stress tests are useful for sedentary patients before they begin an exercise regimen, to evaluate whether exercise is safe for them.
- Stress tests are useful as part of the preoperative work-up for elderly patients and for those with heart risks before they undergo major surgery.

TABLE 15.2 *Preparation for cardiac procedures*

"Nothing by mouth," also known as "nil per os" (NPO)
For many cardiac procedures, you may be directed by your physician not to eat or drink after midnight before the scheduled procedure, including coffee and orange juice. Only a sip of water with routine medications is allowed, and only if permitted by your doctor. Ask your doctor if you can take all your medications, or if you should take only some of them—or even none of them.

Blood thinners and antiplatelet medications
Ask your doctor if you should continue taking blood thinners and antiplatelet medications before surgery. Some invasive procedures may require that you stop taking these medications a few days before the procedure. *Always check with your physician before stopping blood thinners or antiplatelet medications.* In most circumstances, antiplatelet medications should not be discontinued. Sometimes, the physician will choose to stop the oral blood thinner and order an injectable form of blood thinner or admit you to the hospital for intravenous blood thinners to bridge blood thinner treatment and decrease your risk of stroke.

such as acetylsalicylic acid (aspirin) and clopidogrel (Plavix), before a procedure. If you have any questions about how to prepare for a diagnostic test or a surgical procedure, ask your doctor well before the test is scheduled.

CHAPTER 16

Continuous Monitoring Devices

Based on the frequency and severity of your symptoms, your doctor may find it useful to monitor and record your rhythm under various circumstances over a specified time. A Holter monitor is a box about the size of a small tape recorder that can record the heart rhythm over a period of 24 to 48 hours. As long as you are wearing the monitor, your heart rhythm can be effectively recorded. This device is useful in determining if you have an arrhythmia and if so, what type of arrhythmia; the information it provides may also help explain syncopal episodes (passing out or fainting).

When recording over a longer period of time, an event recorder or a loop recorder would be more appropriate. The event recorder records information only while you are attached to the recorder; the device is activated by pressing a button. This means that you must activate the recorder when you feel an arrhythmia or palpitations. A loop recorder records information similar to that recorded by the event recorder, but it may record information before you activate the device and will continue to record information after activation.

An implantable loop recorder (also called an implantable cardiac monitor) can be put in a person for long-term monitoring—up to three years, depending on the device. The monitor is placed under the skin (subcutaneously) while the patient is given local anesthesia. This procedure is considered minor surgery; it is fairly easy to perform and usually does not result in complications.

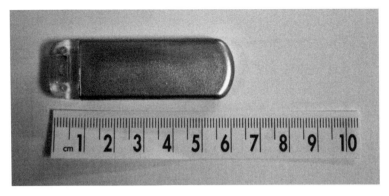

FIGURE 16.1. An implantable loop recorder (or implantable cardiac monitor), which is inserted under the skin through a simple surgical procedure. This device is used to monitor and record electrical activity from your heart.

TABLE 16.1 *Monitors prescribed based on symptom frequency*

Frequency of symptoms	Type of device
Every day	Holter monitor
Once a week	Event recorder, external loop recorder
Once a month	Event recorder, implantable cardiac monitor
Less than once a month	Event recorder, implantable cardiac monitor

An example of an implantable cardiac monitor, or loop recorder, is shown in figure 16.1. Monitoring devices are recommended in part based on frequency of symptoms (see table 16.1). Please talk with your doctor about what kind of monitor is most appropriate for you.

CHAPTER 17

Echocardiogram

An echocardiogram, also called an echo or a cardiac ultrasound, uses sound waves to create images of the heart. The images provided by the echocardiogram are useful to the doctor who is seeking information about your heart's structure and function. This test can reveal your heart's ejection fraction (EF), the presence of leaky or tight (stenotic) valves, weak heart muscles (cardiomyopathies), thick heart muscles (hypertrophy), blood clots or masses in your heart, or fluid in the sac around the heart (the pericardium). The echocardiogram is also useful in showing the presence and location of a heart attack. An echocardiogram machine with an echo (ultrasound) image of the heart seen on the screen is depicted in figure 17.1.

Sometimes this test is performed through the esophagus (called a *transesophageal echocardiogram*), where it is particularly useful in looking for the presence of blood clots in the left atrium. Blood clots may form in the left atrial appendage (a site that is not well visualized by standard echocardiogram but can be clearly visualized by the transesophageal procedure). This test is used frequently in patients who have a history of atrial fibrillation and have not been taking adequate blood thinners or taking blood thinners long enough. If no clot is seen on the transesophageal echocardiogram, it may be safe to proceed with an electrical cardioversion (shock) to convert atrial fibrillation safely.

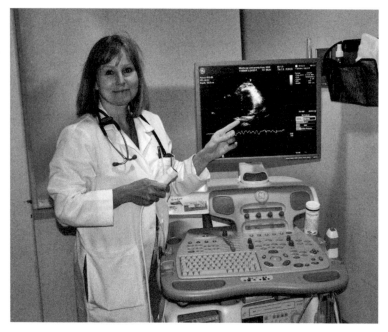

FIGURE 17.1.   An echocardiogram machine demonstrating blood flow throughout the heart.

An echocardiogram can be performed together with a stress test (a stress echocardiogram procedure) to identify the presence of a significantly blocked coronary artery.

An ultrasound probe adapted to one of the catheters can be used for imaging during a catheter ablation procedure. This intra-cardiac echo (ICE) catheter can help visualize internal structures as

TABLE 17.1   *Echocardiogram facts*

- An echocardiogram (also called an echo) is safe: it uses only sound waves.
- An echo can provide useful images of the heart, its valves, its function, and the presence of fluid around the heart or masses in the heart.
- It can help determine the ejection fraction (EF).
- It can be used with a stress test.

well as catheter contact and lesion formation, guide the transseptal procedure, and monitor for pericardial effusion formation (a sign of a perforation) during the procedure. For a summary of key facts about this useful and safe test, see table 17.1.

CHAPTER 18

Computerized Axial Tomography (CT) Angiogram and Cardiac Magnetic Resonance Imaging (MRI)

A test called a CT angiogram may be useful in demonstrating heart function and visualizing the arteries to the heart. A CT angiogram is also helpful in diagnosing coronary artery disease because it is a direct method of looking at the coronary arteries. The heart is constantly moving, making it hard to get a good picture, but CT scanner scientists have compensated for this problem and have developed techniques making it possible to obtain an adequate image of the heart.

With this procedure, you are given contrast dye intravenously and receive an amount of radiation comparable to having a cardiac angiogram. Notify your doctor if you have any known allergies to dye, so he or she can take measures to avoid your having an allergic reaction during the procedure.

Similar to a CT angiogram, cardiac MRI is a test used to take pictures of the heart to diagnose coronary artery disease, assess damage caused by a previous heart attack, and diagnose heart failure as well as valve problems. A cardiac MRI may yield diagnostic information similar to what is produced by a CT angiogram, although visualization of the arteries is limited. This form of MRI is a useful test that usually poses no serious threat to the patient, except for some with a metallic implantable device (such as an implantable defibrillator).

The cardiac MRI is particularly useful at looking for an inherited condition called *arrhythmogenic right ventricular dysplasia* (in which fat deposits are seen within the wall of the right ventricle). Patients with this disorder may be at high risk for sudden cardiac arrest and ventricular tachycardia and should be considered candidates for an implantable cardioverter defibrillator (ICD).

In addition, CT angiography and cardiac MRI may both be useful for visualizing the pulmonary veins and the left atrium (which is useful during an atrial fibrillation ablation).

A variety of imaging techniques exist that can help reveal the heart and its function and structures. Cardiologists and radiologists skilled in using these imaging modalities may help the electrophysiologist gain a better understanding of your heart and help guide the electrophysiologist's interventions.

CHAPTER 19

Cardiac Catheterization, Coronary Angiogram, Left Ventriculogram, Angioplasty, and Stenting

Based on your history and medical condition, your doctor may recommend an invasive procedure called a *cardiac catheterization*. This procedure is performed in a specialized laboratory (called a catheterization laboratory, or cath lab) under x-ray visualization (cinefluoroscopy) by placing catheters (tubes) through sheaths into the blood vessels (artery and/or vein) and threading the catheters into the heart. Patients are generally given sedation before or during the procedure so they feel more comfortable. Contrast dye is administered to visualize structures, and pressures are recorded to determine heart and valve function. *Please tell your doctor if you have a contrast dye allergy or a shellfish allergy prior to the procedure. In addition, you should notify your doctor if you are allergic to latex.*

A cardiac catheterization may have several components. The following are just some of the types of cardiac catheterization procedures that may be performed.

Coronary Angiogram

The coronary arteries and any blockages can be visualized by injecting contrast dye. The type of image obtained from a coronary angiogram is shown in figure 19.1.

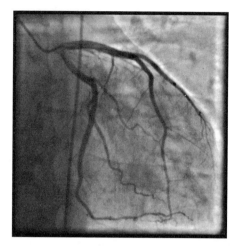

FIGURE 19.1. Visualization of the left coronary artery during a coronary angiogram. A catheter was inserted into the femoral artery in the groin and manipulated around the aorta into the opening of the left coronary artery. Contrast dye was then injected and cinefluoroscopic images were recorded. Additional images and views were recorded to completely image the coronary artery anatomy.

Left Ventriculogram

A catheter is advanced around the aorta and across the aortic valve, and contrast dye is injected into the left ventricle to visualize its function and calculate the ejection fraction (EF).

Percutaneous Coronary Intervention

Percutaneous Coronary Intervention (PCI) refers to an invasive procedure used to treat blockages within the coronary arteries. This procedure may include percutaneous transluminal coronary angioplasty (PTCA), in which a balloon catheter is placed across a coronary artery blockage to open up the occlusion; and stenting, in which a piece of metal mesh, called a *stent,* is deployed at the site to keep the blood vessel open after PTCA. A stent may be made of bare metal or it may be drug coated.

The risks of these procedures are less for the diagnostic studies (coronary angiogram and LV angiogram) and slightly more for the PCI procedures. These risks include bleeding, clot formation, damage to the blood vessels or heart (including perforation), contrast dye reaction (including possible injury to the kidneys), dissection of a blood vessel, coronary artery occlusion, heart attack, heart rhythm abnormality, stroke, cardiac arrest, and death.

After any of these procedures, patients go to a recovery room for monitoring. In the recovery room, the sheaths are removed and pressure is applied to the access sites for 15 to 30 minutes. To prevent bleeding, patients must lie flat for 6 hours or more after these procedures. Occasionally, special tools and devices may be used to help close the blood vessels. Your doctor will explain the test results to you and your family.

....

I had never given much thought to undergoing an angiogram before I had one. Of course I had heard that angiograms were the gold standard for diagnosing cardiovascular disease, but I also knew that they were not routinely performed on patients without a medical reason. I did not have a single symptom to justify an angiogram; no chest pain, no shortness of breath, and a normal stress test the previous year.

After I suddenly collapsed, I was still having trouble comprehending what had happened to me and why I was being told that I was lucky to be alive. In the hospital, when I heard the doctor mention the need for an angiogram that evening, I began to appreciate the significance of what had happened to me. My first thoughts were of my wife's mother, who had died from cardiac disease thirty years ago. I can still remember her describing to me the pain associated with cardiac catheterizations at that time and how she feared having to undergo several such procedures. I was as much concerned about the pain involved in the procedure as I was about what my doctor would find.

My doctor reassured me that it would be a painless procedure and that he would be looking for an explanation of what had happened to me. He thought that it was sudden cardiac arrest, based on my lack of symptoms, and he was hoping that he could place stents in my arteries if he found treatable blockages. If he could not treat me with stents, I would have to be transferred to another hospital for coronary artery bypass grafts. I began to root real hard for the stents.

The next morning was a blur. I recall being wheeled out from my room with wishes of good luck from the wonderful nursing staff and then arriving in an intimidating white room. I was placed on a table and spoke with some very caring people in the room. The doctor came in and once again explained that I could watch the procedure on the monitors next to me, but I politely declined the invitation. I was told that I would feel a warm sensation, and that's the last thing I remember until I woke up to the good news from my doctor that he had found two significant blockages that he was able to treat with stents. The procedure was quick, uneventful, and painless. Even the wound in my groin healed quickly and with minimal discomfort.

Dealing with the stents has been less cumbersome than I would have expected. They are truly a medical miracle. I have no surgical marks on my chest. I sometimes try to feel if they are there, but of course, I don't feel a thing. I have met a surprising number of people who have had stents inserted. One client sent me a get well message addressed to a "two-stenter" from a "three-stenter." I found out that a friend of mine, who happens to be a doctor, is a "six-stenter," as he calls himself with great pride.

With the ability to exercise now and to raise my heart rate, I feel much more confident that the stents are doing their job and that I can live a normal life. My doctors have done their job well. Now it is my job to eat properly, to exercise, to take my medications, and to try to manage stress better. I'm still working on the last one.

CHAPTER 20

T-Wave Alternans (TWA)

T-wave alternans (TWA) is a test that can be performed in your doctor's office or medical facility (table 20.1). This test is typically advised for people who have had a heart attack or other damage to their heart. It can assess their risk for sudden cardiac arrest related to ventricular tachycardia or ventricular fibrillation. With TWA, you are attached by electrodes to computerized equipment and undergo a stress test. An intravenous line is inserted and continuous ECG monitoring is performed. The computer analyzes your heart rhythm for a scientific phenomenon called *microvolt T-wave alternans*.

An abnormal or inconclusive test may show the doctor that you are at risk for ventricular tachycardia or ventricular fibrillation (sudden cardiac arrest). The doctor may then refer you for an electrophysiology study to determine whether an implantable defibrillator would be beneficial for you.

TABLE 20.1 *T-wave alternans (TWA)*

- TWA is a test to determine your risk for ventricular tachycardia.
- It is not useful if you are in atrial fibrillation.

CHAPTER 21

Electrophysiology Study (EP Study)

The electrophysiology study (EP study) is a crucial procedure for identifying heart rhythm problems. This invasive test is typically administered to patients who are thought to have some type of arrhythmia. The procedure is performed in a specially equipped room called the EP lab, using specialized stimulating equipment and recording technology to assess the heart's electrical system (figure 21.1). The electrophysiologist (heart rhythm specialist) may choose to use mapping equipment to locate the area where the abnormal heart rhythm is originating. For this procedure, you must have specialized pads placed on your chest and upper back (which can be used to shock you if necessary), and an intravenous line must be inserted. Continuous heart monitoring is essential throughout this procedure.

During the EP study, catheters are guided through blood vessels into the heart using an x-ray technique called *fluoroscopy imaging*. The catheters are placed through the veins, arteries, or both up into the chambers of the heart. Electrical signals are recorded directly from the heart. From this electrophysiology (EP) catheter, the doctor is able to pace (stimulate) your heart at a faster rate than normal and take recordings of the signals. This test can reveal if you need a pacemaker or a defibrillator. In addition, this test can help to identify the precise type of rapid heart rhythm (tachycardia) that you have. Sometimes during this test, the doctor decides to utilize another procedure, called catheter ablation, in which the rhythm

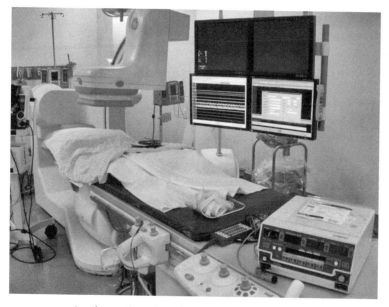

FIGURE 21.1.   An electrophysiology laboratory. A typical lab consists of a procedural table; x-ray imaging equipment; computerized monitoring, recording, analyzing, and electrical stimulating equipment; and a defibrillator (shocking device; see figure 21.2). The box in the lower righthand corner is used for delivering radiofrequency energy during a catheter ablation procedure to cure rhythm problems. Some laboratories also have a separate control room where the doctor or staff may sit to pace (stimulate) the heart and induce arrhythmias.

is mapped and treated with energy such as radio waves to cure the abnormality.

The reasons for having an EP study include diagnosing unexplained rhythm problems, passing out (syncope), or unexplained palpitations or light-headedness; performing a curative procedure such as catheter ablation; or determining whether there is a need for implantable device therapy (see table 21.1). Appendix A presents a more in-depth list of the indications for an EP study obtained from a consensus statement from the American College of Cardiology, American Heart Association, and Heart Rhythm Society guidelines.

TABLE 21.1   *When do you need an EP study?*

To diagnose unexplained rhythm problems
To determine the cause of fainting or blacking out (syncope)
To diagnose unexplained palpitations, light-headedness, or dizziness
    (presyncope)
To cure a rhythm problem with a catheter ablation procedure
To determine if you need a pacemaker or defibrillator

Patients need to understand the risks, benefits, and alternatives to this invasive procedure. The risks include bleeding, clot formation, perforation, heart attack, cardiac arrest, stroke, and death. Major complications are relatively uncommon. Your doctor may provide some sedation during the procedure to make you more comfortable. You may feel the sensation of a fast heart rate, which may be similar to your symptoms of palpitations or flutters in the chest. This procedure is performed in a carefully controlled setting in the presence of the doctor and qualified and trained support staff.

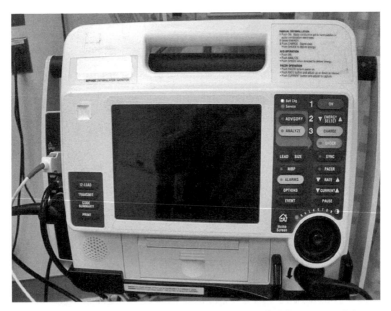

FIGURE 21.2.   A cardiac monitor with pacing and defibrillation capabilities.

While undergoing such a procedure, you may be given a shock by the doctor if necessary to terminate a significant arrhythmia such as ventricular tachycardia or fibrillation. When a shock is unsynchronized, it is called *defibrillation*; when it is synchronized it is called *cardioversion*. An external defibrillator, which can be used to shock a patient out of tachycardia, is pictured in figure 21.2. As with any test, it is important to communicate with the facility's staff and let them know if you are experiencing symptoms such as palpitations, chest pain, or any discomfort.

CHAPTER 22

Tilt Table Test

....

A tilt table test is a very simple, noninvasive test used to investigate light-headedness, dizziness, and loss of consciousness (syncope). The purpose of this test is to try to replicate your symptoms and potentially provoke a syncopal episode. A positive test result may show a drop in blood pressure with or without a significant change in heart rate.

During this procedure, you lie down on a specialized table that can be tilted nearly upright at an angle prescribed by the doctor (usually 60–80 degrees) for up to 45 minutes (figure 22.1). Electrodes are placed on your chest, and an intravenous line is put in a vein. Occasionally, a medicine may be infused into the intravenous line to elicit a positive test result—an abnormal heart rate or rhythm and possible blood vessel response in which your blood pressure may drop and your heart rate slow down. This reaction is called neurocardiogenic, or vasovagal, syncope. If this reaction occurs, the table will be adjusted downward, you will be placed flat, and your symptoms will normally subside within seconds. If your heart rate drops significantly and symptoms such as unresponsiveness or persistent slow heart rate (bradycardia) occur, you will be treated immediately with medications or the doctor may choose to pace (stimulate) your heart through specialized pacing pads.

Many patients have a misconception that the tilt table test is one in which the patient's head is tilted back. Some patients come in for the test thinking it is going to be much like a ride at an amuse-

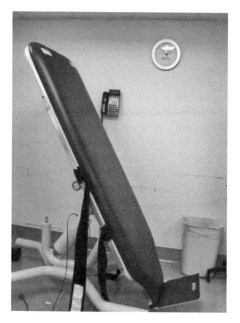

FIGURE 22.1. An upright tilt table, which is used to elicit syncope in susceptible patients. The patient is fastened to the table, and it is brought nearly upright in order to evaluate the patient's heart rate and blood pressure response to an upright position. An intravenous medication may be administered to facilitate the test.

ment park (the Tilt-a-Whirl). This test is more like standing straight upright for a prolonged period in the same spot, as though you were waiting in a long line. The tilt table test is relatively safe and is unlikely to result in any serious complications. Frequent and clear communication between the patient and the staff is essential.

PART SIX

Procedures and Medications for Treating Heart Problems

CHAPTER 23

Catheter Ablation

....

Many rhythm problems can be treated with catheter ablation, which is often performed as an extension of an electrophysiology (EP) study. In catheter ablation, a long thin medical device called an ablation catheter is inserted by hand through a blood vessel and then is guided into the heart using x-ray or mapping equipment to find and treat abnormal rhythms. Occasionally, the ablation catheter can be remotely controlled using more complex equipment.

Heart conditions that can be treated with ablation procedures are summarized in table 23.1. Once the site that is sustaining an arrhythmia is identified, energy is applied through the catheter to its tip, as radio waves or another form of energy, to destroy (ablate) the abnormal rhythm. A generator used to deliver radiofrequency energy to ablate cardiac tissue is shown in figure 23.1. The risks of EP study are described in chapter 21; there are also risks in catheter ablation, including an increased risk of heart perforation and damage to the heart's normal conduction system, potentially requiring a pacemaker implant (although this is a rare complication).

More difficult ablation procedures are often left sided and may require additional equipment such as intracardiac echocardiography (ICE) and a 3-D mapping system. The 3-D mapping equipment is used to identify the type of arrhythmia and assist in finding where the arrhythmia originates. It can also track the location of each ablation that is applied to the heart. Some complex ablation procedures may require the use of blood thinners, temporary use of an

TABLE 23.1   *Heart conditions treated by ablation procedures*

Easier to treat	More difficult to treat
Typical atrial flutter	Ventricular tachycardia
AV node reentry	Atrial fibrillation
AV node ablation	Atrial tachycardia
	Wolff-Parkinson-White syndrome

artificial airway, and general anesthesia. Your doctor will discuss his or her recommendations if you are diagnosed with an arrhythmia that might benefit from a catheter ablation procedure.

The anticipated success rates for specific types of ablation procedures are presented in table 23.2. Success rates differ based on physician experience, in this case the number of procedures the physician has performed and how long he or she has practiced elec-

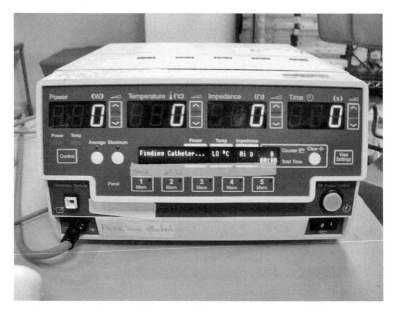

FIGURE 23.1.   A catheter ablation radiofrequency generator. The generator is hooked to a cable and then connected to a steerable ablation catheter (which is inserted in the person). Grounding patches are also placed on the person as part of the procedure.

TABLE 23.2   *Anticipated success rates of types of catheter ablation procedures*

Ablation type	Anticipated success

Supraventricular tachycardia:
  Atrial flutter
  Atrial tachycardia
  AV node
  AV node reentrant tachycardia
  Wolff-Parkinson-White syndrome
	90 percent or greater

Atrial fibrillation	50 to 85 percent
Ventricular tachycardia from coronary artery disease	50 to 75 percent
Focal ventricular tachycardia	90 percent or greater

Source: Derived from T. J. Cohen, *Practical Electrophysiology,* 2nd ed. (Malvern, PA: HMP Communications, 2009), p. 99.

trophysiology. In general, the greater the physician's experience, the greater the success rate. Ablation of garden variety ventricular tachycardia is more complicated than ablation of garden variety supraventricular tachycardia (excluding atrial fibrillation, which is a specific type of supraventricular tachycardia). Success rates for ablation of supraventricular tachycardia are typically greater than 90 percent if treated properly. Success rates for atrial fibrillation ablation depend on the duration and type of heart disease; rates of cure range from 50 to 85 percent. More than one procedure may be required to achieve success from atrial fibrillation ablation. Ventricular tachycardia that is due to coronary artery disease or a heart attack is ablated with a success rate of between 50 and 75 percent. Certain types of ventricular tachycardias that begin from a specific site in a more normal heart have a very high cure rate of more than 90 percent if treated properly.

CHAPTER 24

Electrical Cardioversion and Defibrillation

In performing a cardioversion or defibrillation procedure, a physician is working to convert an abnormal heart rhythm to a normal heart rhythm (see table 24.1). Cardioversion can be performed either electrically or chemically. Electrical cardioversion, often thought of as "shocking" someone, is performed with a defibrillator (a shocking device). Cardioversion and defibrillation are essentially the same procedure with the same goal, except that cardioversion is performed in more stable rapid heart rhythms by synchronizing shock delivery to the peak of the QRS complex seen on the ECG (see chapter 14). This synchronization process takes more time than unsynchronized shock delivery (defibrillation). When the heart rhythm is too rapid and chaotic (as it is with ventricular fibrillation) and time is of the essence (as with unstable ventricular tachycardia), defibrillation is performed.

When a person needs electrical cardioversion or defibrillation outside the hospital's electrophysiology laboratory, paddles placed directly on the chest may be used as well as patches (or pads). Proper placement of external paddles while administering a shock is demonstrated in figure 24.1. When patches are used, electrical energy is delivered from the defibrillator through the patches to the chest. When people undergo this procedure in the electrophysiology lab, they are attached by special wires and patches to a standard external defibrillator, which is different from an implantable cardioverter defibrillator (discussed in chapter 27). When this procedure is elec-

TABLE 24.1 *Electrical cardioversion and defibrillation*

- Electrical cardioversion and defibrillation are useful for breaking fast rhythms
- They are used to terminate (convert)
    - atrial fibrillation
    - atrial flutter
    - ventricular fibrillation
    - ventricular flutter
    - any rapid rhythm that does not respond to standard drugs and is not stable, such as when the patient is semiconscious or unconscious or has a low blood pressure

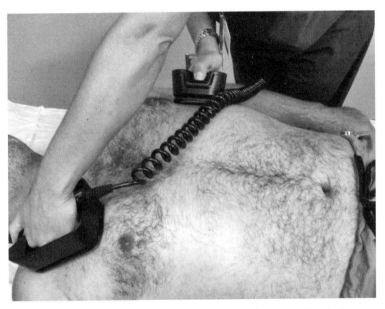

FIGURE 24.1. How a health care provider would administer electrical energy via external paddles to a person with a life-threatening arrhythmia to restore a normal cardiac rhythm.

tive (rather than an emergency), patients are sedated. An external defibrillator is used to shock the patient out of rapid heart rhythms in the upper chamber of the heart (atrial fibrillation and atrial flutter) as well as to treat very serious rhythms from the lower chambers (ventricular tachycardia and ventricular fibrillation).

To perform chemical cardioversion, the doctor may use medications known as antiarrhythmic drugs to help convert certain arrhythmias (such as atrial fibrillation and atrial flutter) into normal rhythms. In general, however, delivering electrical energy by means of defibrillation (or electrical cardioversion) is the treatment of choice when patients have symptoms and are not stable. For a review of some key factors regarding electrical cardioversion and defibrillation, see table 24.1.

CHAPTER 25

Heart Medications

Prescription medications are an important treatment option for patients with heart rhythm problems. They are useful in treating risk factors of heart disease such as high blood pressure and high cholesterol. Early treatment with medication can lower a person's risk of developing a heart attack and subsequent sudden cardiac arrest. This chapter discusses many of the drugs taken by people with heart disease or by people who are at risk for heart disease.

The following five general principles about medications are applicable to most people with heart disease or risk factors for heart disease. First, certain medications, such as beta blockers, are useful in treating a number of different conditions such as high blood pressure (hypertension), coronary artery disease, and congestive heart failure. Your doctor may prescribe your medication for one or more of these conditions. Second, you should pay close attention to instructions on how to take your medications. Instructions include the timing (when and how often) and dosage of the medication as well as whether you should take the medication with meals. If you miss one pill, take the next regularly scheduled pill. In addition, some medications are less active if a person has eaten grapefruit or grapefruit juice or has taken nonsteroidal anti-inflammatory drugs (also called NSAIDs) such as ibuprofen. You may be instructed not to consume grapefruit or grapefruit juice or not to take NSAIDs while you are on these medications. *Follow the instructions for any prescribed medication. Following medical instructions (called* medical compliance*) is essential to achieve the drug's desired effects.*

Third, potential side effects and potential drug interactions should be covered in a discussion between you and your doctor or pharmacist before you start taking the drug. Bring any significant side effect to your doctor's attention. The more medications used, the more likely the side effects. Fourth, notify your doctor before stopping *any* medication. Finally, report any suspected drug allergies to your doctor. Keep a list of your current medications and drug allergies in your wallet at all times and show the list to any health care provider you consult.

Heart Rhythm (Antiarrhythmic) Drugs

A number of medicines are prescribed to treat heart rhythm problems and minimize complications associated with arrhythmias. Two major categories of medicines used to treat arrhythmias are antiarrhythmic drugs and anticoagulants (also known as blood thinners). The American College of Cardiology, American Heart Association, and the Heart Rhythm Society review ongoing research and collaborate with one another in making recommendations for safe and effective management of patients with arrhythmias. In 2003 the guidelines for supraventricular arrhythmias were updated, and in 2006 the guidelines for atrial fibrillation and ventricular arrhythmias management were updated (see the bibliography for a list of current expert sources for arrhythmia management).

Antiarrhythmic drugs work by altering the electrical signals of the heart. Common heart rhythm medications that may be prescribed by your doctor are listed in table 25.1. Each of these medications has a version that may be taken by mouth (orally ingested); an intravenous (IV) version of the drug may also exist. The most common antiarrhythmic drugs are the beta blockers, which are very useful in controlling the heart rate as well as treating patients with coronary artery disease, congestive heart failure, and high blood

TABLE 25.1 *Common heart rhythm (antiarrhythmic) medications and their effects*

Medicine	Effects	Comments
Beta blocker	Slows pulse (treats SVT*); lowers blood pressure, helps treat heart failure and coronary artery disease	Avoid in patients with asthma; can cause impotence, depression
Calcium channel blocker	Slows pulse (treats SVT); lowers blood pressure	Not as good as a beta blocker if you have coronary artery disease
Amiodarone	Best drug treatment for ventricular tachycardia and atrial fibrillation or flutter	Many potential side effects: can affect thyroid, liver, lungs; requires follow-up every three months; ventricular tachycardia (proarrhythmia) is a rare complication
Sotalol	Less effective than amiodarone for ventricular tachycardia and atrial fibrillation or flutter	Can bring on or worsen ventricular tachycardia (proarrhythmia)
Dofetilide	Can treat atrial fibrillation or flutter	Can bring on or worsen ventricular tachycardia (proarrhythmia)
Dronedarone	Can treat atrial fibrillation or flutter	Amiodarone-like drug with fewer side effects
Mexiletine	Even less effective than sotalol for ventricular tachycardia	Does not worsen ventricular tachycardia; can cause confusion, dizziness, numbness, and tingling
Flecainide	Can treat SVT and atrial fibrillation	Can bring on ventricular tachycardia (proarrhythmia)
Propafenone	Can treat SVT and atrial fibrillation	Can bring on ventricular tachycardia (proarrhythmia)

*SVT = supraventricular tachycardia.

pressure. In addition to beta blockers, patients may be prescribed daily blood thinners, such as warfarin.

Another category of medications that help control the rate of supraventricular arrhythmias are calcium channel blockers. Note that dietary calcium intake or calcium supplements do not interfere with calcium channel blockers.

More potent antiarrhythmic medications include amiodarone, dofetilide, dronedarone, sotalol, propafenone, mexiletine, and flecainide. Ibutilide, a drug used to treat atrial fibrillation and atrial flutter, is not listed in table 25.1 because it is available only in an intravenous form; it has no orally digested version. The most consequential side effect for heart rhythm medications is proarrhythmia, which is a more serious rhythm disturbance than the original problem. A type of ventricular tachycardia called *torsades de pointes* may be brought on by some of these medications in some people.

Dronedarone (an amiodarone-like drug) was the most recent antiarrhythmic drug approved by the United States Food and Drug Administration (FDA) for the treatment of atrial fibrillation. This drug is similar to amiodarone but has less severe toxicity and side effects. In particular, dronedarone does not have the lung, liver, and thyroid toxicity that sometimes occurs with amiodarone.

If, based on the expert guidelines, your doctor has prescribed any of these medications for you, then you may be asked to see your doctor more frequently for follow-up to avoid complications.

Other Heart-Related Drugs

Other medications used to treat common heart conditions such as coronary artery disease, congestive heart failure, arrhythmias, and hypertension are detailed in table 25.2.

Drugs used to treat coronary artery disease

Sudden cardiac arrest is often the result of ventricular tachycardia or ventricular fibrillation that arises from injured areas of the heart.

TABLE 25.2   *Other common heart drugs*

Coronary artery disease medications

Nitroglycerine: Used to treat chest pain (called angina) from coronary artery disease. Can lower blood pressure. Should not be taken by patients using sildenafil (Viagra).

Beta blockers: A medication that blocks the beta-adrenergic receptors in the heart. As a result, this medication blocks the effects of adrenaline. Used to limit the workload of the heart. May also slow down the heart rate and help lower blood pressure. Side effects include exacerbation of asthma, drop in blood pressure, depression, and impotence.

Antiplatelet Medications

Acetylsalicylic acid (aspirin): Used to help prevent a heart attack. It is also helpful for patients having a heart attack to chew an aspirin.

Clopidogrel (Plavix): Used with acetylsalicylic acid (aspirin) after placement of a stent to prevent the stent and coronary artery from occluding.

Lipid-lowering Drugs

HMG-CoA reductase inhibitors (statins): Used to prevent cholesterol buildup in the coronary arteries. Can also prevent the inflammatory response that could cause atheromatous plaques to rupture in the heart and precipitate a heart attack. Side effects include muscle and liver injury.

Niacin (nicotinic acid), cholestyramine, gemfibrozil, clofibrate: Used to treat high cholesterol and high triglycerides.

Heart failure drugs

Angiotensin-converting enzyme (ACE) inhibitors: Used to help improve the heart's function. May vasodilate the blood vessels and lower blood pressure, making it easier for the failing heart to pump blood. It may adversely affect the kidneys and cause a cough in some people.

Angiotensin II receptor blockers (ARBs): Used to help improve the heart's function. May vasodilate the blood vessels and lower blood pressure, making it easier for the failing heart to pump blood. May adversely affect the kidneys.

Beta blockers (see "Coronary artery disease medications" *above):* Can improve heart function in patients with heart failure. Note that some medications act by blocking both alpha (see "Antihypertensive medications" below) and beta receptors. One such drug, carvedilol, blocks the alpha-1 receptor as well as beta receptors.

(*continued*)

TABLE 25.2 *continued*

Digitalis: May make a weak heart pump stronger. May be useful if heart failure does not improve with ACE inhibitors or ARBs. Side effects include worsening heart rhythm problems and yellow vision. Dosage should be reduced in people with heart failure and kidney failure.

Diuretics (fluid pills): Used to eliminate excess fluids in patients with heart failure. May affect kidney function.

Note: ACE inhibitors or ARBs plus a beta blocker fulfill the AHA's Get with the Guidelines heart failure program for treating congestive heart failure.

Anticoagulants (blood thinners)

Warfarin (Coumadin): Decreases risk of stroke in patients with atrial fibrillation and stroke risk factors. The main risk of warfarin is bleeding. The effects are monitored by an INR blood test, which monitors your blood thinner's effect on clotting (coagulation). Green leafy vegetables and other substances that contain vitamin K may lower your INR (blood thinner level) with this medication. The addition of blood thinner to acetylsalicylic acid (aspirin) and clopidogrel (Plavix) may increase the risk of bleeding and bruising. ***Please talk to your doctor about all your medications and your diet before starting warfarin.***

Antihypertensive medications (blood pressure medications)

These medications can have additive effects on the lowering of blood pressure.

Beta blockers. See "Heart failure drugs" above

Alpha blockers: Block alpha-adrenergic receptors (therefore blocking noradrenaline). There are two types of alpha receptors (alpha 1 and alpha 2). These medications can be used to treat prostate enlargement (benign prostatic hypertrophy), Raynaud disease, and high blood pressure.

Combined alpha and beta blockers: May block both the alpha and beta receptors and may be useful in treating high blood pressure as well as heart failure.

Calcium channel blockers: Block the calcium channel receptors. May help lower blood pressure and may also slow down the heart rate. It is important to stay well hydrated and eat fruits and vegetables when taking this medication to avoid constipation as a side effect.

ACE inhibitors. See "Heart failure drugs" above

ARBs. See "Heart failure drugs" above

These injuries may be a result of scarring from a prior heart attack or may occur during sudden cardiac arrest if the person is having a heart attack at the same time. The buildup of fatty deposits such as cholesterol in the coronary arteries (the condition called atherosclerosis) followed by plaque rupture is one common cause of heart attacks. HMG-CoA reductase inhibitors (called statins) are a class of drugs that block not only the buildup of cholesterol but also the inflammatory process that can lead to plaque rupture and subsequent coronary artery occlusion. Other drugs, such as cholestyramine, niacin (nicotinic acid), gemfibrozil, and clofibrate, are used to treat high cholesterol and high triglyceride levels, but these drugs are typically less effective than the statins, especially in patients with known coronary artery disease.

Acetylsalicylic acid (aspirin) is useful in preventing the buildup of platelets around the ruptured plaque and minimizing this inflammatory process, thereby preventing acute coronary artery occlusion. In people who have a stent to treat occlusion, antiplatelet agents including acetylsalicylic acid and a thienopyridine such as clopidogrel (Plavix) are useful in preventing the blood vessel from occluding again. Beta blockers are used to block the effects of adrenaline (by blocking beta receptors in the heart muscle) and to decrease the workload of the heart; they are also useful in preventing ischemia (lack of blood flow to the heart muscle) in people with coronary artery disease. Nitroglycerin can be used sublingually (under the tongue) or topically (in paste or patch form) and can help vasodilate the blood vessels and improve blood flow to the heart muscle. It may be useful in treating chest pain from lack of blood flow (and oxygen) to the heart, a condition called *angina* or *angina pectoris*.

Drugs used to treat atrial fibrillation and atrial flutter

Blood thinners such as warfarin (Coumadin) are used to prevent stroke in people with conditions such as atrial fibrillation and atrial flutter. In patients with atrial fibrillation, structurally normal hearts, and no major risk factors for stroke, acetylsalicylic acid may be useful for stroke prevention. Adding antiplatelet medications such as acetylsalicylic acid and clopidogrel to the drug regimen for patients taking the anticoagulant warfarin may increase the risk of bleeding and bruising. Heart rate control can be achieved with beta blockers or calcium channel blockers. The antiarrhythmic drugs dronedarone, amiodarone, sotalol, dofetilide, propafenone, and flecainide, which are useful in treating atrial fibrillation, are discussed earlier in this chapter.

Drugs used to treat ventricular tachycardia and ventricular fibrillation

The principal way to treat nonreversible or recurrent ventricular tachycardia or ventricular fibrillation (the causes of sudden cardiac arrest) is with a device (an ICD). However, frequent and recurrent episodes, even in patients with an ICD, require treatment with drug therapy to suppress the arrhythmia and prevent frequent shocks from the device. Drugs such as mexiletine, sotalol, and amiodarone may all be useful in preventing ventricular tachycardia and ventricular fibrillation (see table 25.1). Sotalol and dofetilide have a higher chance of causing proarrhythmia than the other medications. Amiodarone may be more effective than the rest but has the greatest toxicity. Dronedarone is the most recently approved drug to treat atrial fibrillation and atrial flutter. It has amiodarone-like properties with fewer reported side effects. Its utility in treating ventricular tachycardia and ventricular fibrillation remains to be determined. Mexiletine is probably the least effective but it has a low incidence of proarrhythmia and is usually well tolerated.

Drugs used to treat heart failure

According to the American Heart Association's Get with the Guidelines heart failure program, heart failure should be treated with a beta blocker plus an angiotensin-converting enzyme (ACE) inhibitor or angiotensin II receptor blocker (ARB) unless the patient cannot tolerate those medications. The weakened heart tries to beat faster and thereby puts greater strain on the heart. Beta blockers work by blocking beta receptors in the heart, allowing it to beat slower while also lowering blood pressure, thereby conserving vital cardiac energy. ACE inhibitors and ARB medications work by vasodilating blood vessels and lowering blood pressure. They help to decrease the amount of work that the heart needs to perform to pump blood. If those drugs are unacceptable, alternative drugs exist. These include other vasodilators such as hydralazine and isosorbide dinitrate.

Water pills, called diuretics, are useful in removing excess fluid that builds up in the body as a result of ineffective pumping of blood by a weakened or diseased heart. These drugs may alter the body's electrolytes (such as potassium) and on occasion can cause arrhythmias. If a problem is suspected, your blood should be tested for an electrolyte abnormality. Digitalis may help to increase the heart muscle's ability to contract, especially if ACE inhibitors or ARBs fail to improve heart failure symptoms. If the blood level of digitalis is too high, arrhythmias may occur. A digitalis blood-level test is used to monitor digitalis blood levels and to prevent or detect toxicity.

In summary, you should know the name, indication (reason for taking), and dosing instructions for all your medications, and you should understand what the common and uncommon side effects are and what the symptoms of these side effects might be. If you feel you are experiencing a side effect, notify your doctor. In fact, if you have any questions related to your medicines, including how and how often to take them, ask your doctor. Although your cardiologist may be taking care of your heart, you are probably seeing other physicians who are also involved in your care. *Bring a list of your medications when visiting any of your physicians.*

PART SEVEN

Devices for Treating Heart Problems

CHAPTER 26

Pacemakers

....

A pacemaker is a device about the size of a half dollar that is typically implanted in the chest and attached to at least one wire, which is threaded to the heart through a vein in the chest. This device is very helpful to people with slow rhythm problems (bradycardias). When the bradycardia is significant or results in serious symptoms, a pacemaker may be indicated. The specific problems encountered by a patient (such as symptoms), as well as any diagnosed heart rhythm problems, make up the indications that determine the need for a procedure or device. A doctor is likely to recommend a pacemaker for people who have symptoms such as light-headedness, dizziness, and syncope attributable to bradycardia. A pacemaker can help regulate the rate and rhythm of the heart.

In 2008 the American College of Cardiology, the American Heart Association, and the Heart Rhythm Society updated the indications for cardiac implantable devices. The indications for pacemaker therapy are listed in appendix B (see also table 26.1). You may want to discuss this list with your doctor and ask him or her to explain which pacemaker indication or indications you have. If you are not sure why a pacemaker has been recommended for you, you should feel free to ask questions and even consider getting a second opinion.

The pacemaker (figure 26.1) is connected to a wire that may be attached to the heart with a screw or wedged into the heart with tiny, soft barbs (figure 26.2). Before the procedure, you will most

TABLE 26.1   *When do you need a pacemaker?*

- If you have slow heart rhythms with symptoms
- If you have advanced heart blocks
- To prevent or treat some rapid rhythms and vasovagal syncope
- To treat heart failure by pacing the right and left ventricles synchronously (called biventricular pacing)

likely be asked to be NPO (not eat or drink for 6 to 8 hours prior to surgery). Prior to any procedure, inform your doctor of any medications you are taking, especially any blood thinners. Pacemaker implantation requires an overnight stay in the hospital so that the patient can be assessed the next day for any postoperative complications. To prevent an infection, you will receive an antibiotic (usually through an IV line) before or during the procedure and will be

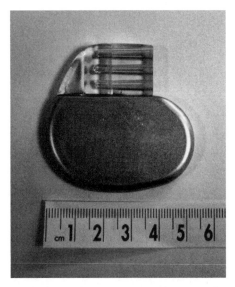

FIGURE 26.1.   A pacemaker pulse generator used to treat slow heart rhythms. One, two, or three leads may be attached to the device depending on the number of heart chambers that are required to receive pacing therapy. The generator shown has three places to connect pacing leads and may be used to help synchronize the right and left ventricles (biventricular pacing).

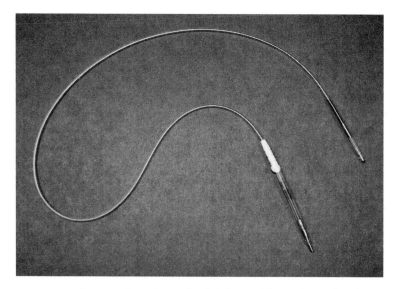

FIGURE 26.2. A pacemaker wire, or lead, is inserted into a heart chamber and then connected to a pacemaker, which is usually implanted in the upper chest, underneath the skin.

required to continue taking an oral antibiotic for a few days after any surgery to implant a device.

During the procedure, the doctor will make a small incision (usually in the upper chest), and the lead or leads will be threaded down to the heart, where they will be able to sense your heart rhythm and provide pacing if your heart rate is slow. Your doctor will determine how many leads you will require. The pacemaker also has the capability to record abnormally fast rhythms.

Your doctor will discuss with you the risks associated with device implantation. They include clot formation, vascular damage or perforation, infection, dislodgment of the lead, and device malfunction. Depending on how the doctor implants the device, there may also be a risk of a collapsed lung. Major complications such as a heart attack, stroke, or death are rare. Although these risks may seem overwhelming, this procedure is relatively safe.

You may have some limitations for 6 weeks following surgery

with respect to exercise and lifting, but in general you will be able to return to your normal daily activities. If you notice any fever or discolored discharge, swelling, or excessive pain at the incision site, contact your doctor's office immediately. These can be symptoms of an infection. Normal follow-up includes a two-week wound check and follow-up device checks at approximately two months, six months, and every six months thereafter. Typically, a pacemaker lasts about eight years (see chapters 31 and 32).

For more details about pacemakers, please refer to appendix B. If there are terms or concepts that you do not understand, ask your doctor about them. (See also chapter 30.)

Implantable Cardioverter Defibrillators (ICDs)

Question: True or false: You cannot use a microwave if you have an ICD (or defibrillator).
Answer: False. Patients with these devices can use a microwave safely.

ICDs were developed in the early 1980s and are very similar to pacemakers. Just like a pacemaker, an ICD consists of a pulse generator and a lead or leads. To treat rapid rhythms completely, these devices must be able to terminate rapid rhythms (ventricular tachycardia and ventricular fibrillation). To do this, ICDs deliver high-voltage DC energy, and therefore they require more electrical circuitry and battery power and are considerably larger than a pacemaker. They are the size of a deck of cards rather than the size of a half dollar. In general, the lead that is used in an ICD to cardiovert, or defibrillate, is slightly thicker and stiffer than a standard pacemaker lead.

ICDs help regulate both fast rhythms (tachycardias) and slow rhythms (bradycardias). Simply put, ICDs monitor the heart rate, and if it is greater than a predetermined (or programmed) value, the ICD may deliver therapy to treat the arrhythmia. Ventricular tachycardia or ventricular fibrillation may be treated by the delivery of a shock (defibrillation) or rapid pacing (also called *antitachycardia pacing*). This ability to deliver a shock to the heart to terminate tachycardias is one important difference between an ICD and a simple pacemaker.

A patient might benefit from an ICD in various scenarios (see table 27.1). These types of devices are indicated in patients who have experienced a sudden cardiac arrest, especially if the cause is not reversible. ICDs are also indicated in patients with ventricular tachycardia, whether spontaneous or induced during an EP study. In patients with unexplained loss of consciousness (syncope) and heart disease, an ICD is often very helpful. There are prophylactic indications for these devices (also called *primary prevention* because the person has not yet had an event), such as for patients with mild to moderate congestive heart failure and an ejection fraction of 35 percent or less. Patients who have had a prior heart attack (myocardial infarction) and have an ejection fraction of 30 percent or less may also benefit from ICD therapy. For a more complete list of ICD indications derived in part from the American College of Cardiology, American Heart Association, and Heart Rhythm Society guidelines, see appendix C. If you have been referred for an ICD implant, you may want to discuss this list with your doctor and ask him or her to explain which ICD indication or indications you have. If you are not sure why an ICD has been recommended for you, you should feel free to ask questions and even consider getting a second opinion. Typically an ICD lasts about six years. (See also chapters 30, 31, and 32.)

An ICD pulse generator is about the size of a large pager or a deck of cards (see figure 27.1). The procedure for implanting an ICD is very similar to that for implanting a pacemaker. The increase

TABLE 27.1 *When do you need a defibrillator?*

- After cardiac arrest due to an arrhythmia
- If you have symptomatic ventricular tachycardia or ventricular fibrillation
- If you have ventricular tachycardia or ventricular fibrillation induced during an EP study
- If you have loss of consciousness (syncope) and structural heart disease
- If you have an EF of 35 percent or less and mild to moderate heart failure
- If you have an EF of 30 percent or less and a prior heart attack

---

in size and complexity of the pulse generator, and the increased size and stiffness of the high-voltage ICD lead carry a slightly higher risk of complications from implanting an ICD compared with implanting a pacemaker. Many of the risks involved in ICD surgery are the same, however, and include clot formation, vascular damage or perforation, infection, lead dislodgment, device malfunction, heart attack, stroke, and death. The ICD recovery period is also similar to that of a pacemaker. Normal follow-up includes a two-week wound check and device checks at approximately two months, six months, and every six months thereafter. People who receive an ICD are instructed to call their doctor's office if they receive one shock; if they receive two or more shocks, it is important that they be seen by a physician as soon as possible.

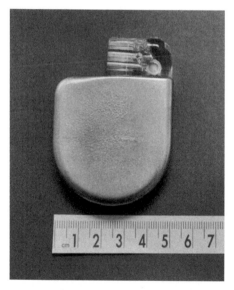

FIGURE 27.1. An implantable cardioverter defibrillator (ICD) pulse generator, which is used to treat rapid rhythms from the lower chamber of the heart, called ventricular tachycardia or ventricular fibrillation. Note that the specific type of ICD shown in this figure is a biventricular device (see chapter 28).

On Sunday morning, I finished my usual morning swim at the local Y and headed down to the marina to clean my boat. The traffic was stop and go, so I lit another cigarette and sipped my coffee as I began the hour-long drive. Little did I know that on this day, my life would change forever.

I had been working on the boat for several hours and was almost finished when I suddenly began to feel extremely tired. My hands were cramping up, and I felt tightness in my throat. I left the boat to lie down on the grass until I felt able to walk a few yards to a restaurant, where I drank a few glasses of orange juice. Still feeling weak, and totally clueless about what was happening, I left the marina and drove home. My hands were still cramping, and I was just not feeling right. I wondered if inhaling fumes from the acetone cleaner was making me feel sick. I arrived home exhausted. I showered and went to sleep, certain that I would be fine in the morning. But I wasn't. Next morning I noticed that every time I climbed a flight of stairs, I felt tightness in my throat and was short of breath. Now I was frightened. Could I be having a heart attack?

I got into the car and drove the few blocks to my internist's office. He immediately arranged for a stress test, but a minute into the test, I was told I needed an angiogram. Then panic set in. "This can't be real," I thought, "I'm a healthy guy." But the angiogram revealed serious blockages in my coronary arteries, and I was told that I would have to have triple bypass surgery. I was shocked, scared, and angry. But then reality set in, and I knew I had had a heart attack.

I was relieved when my surgeon told me that the surgery had gone well. I would have a second chance. But I was also depressed. I had to change my lifestyle in so many ways. I was prescribed a heart-healthy diet and told that I had to stop smoking cigarettes. I entered a cardiac rehab program and slowly regained my strength. But I couldn't kick the cigarette habit. I continued smoking in secret, hiding cigarettes in the trunk of my car and driving with the car windows open even in the coldest weather to conceal the odor of the smoke from my family. The doctor had said that I survived the heart attack because collateral blood vessels had formed from my daily swim. I started to swim again. I thought that I could continue smoking as long as I kept up the swimming. I was wrong.

Two years after my bypass surgery, I underwent a stress test and experienced a brief episode of ventricular tachycardia. After that I went for an electrophysiology study, which showed that I needed an implantable defibrillator. Six weeks after I received the implant, I felt the device go off. It has gone off three more times since. Each time the defibrillator responded appropriately by shocking my heart back to its normal rhythm—thereby saving my life. I felt fine after each shock. There was no warning beforehand. I am grateful to my doctor and thankful for my defibrillator. It gives me hope that I can live to a ripe old age. After all, it saved my life four times. Oh yes, one more thing—I finally stopped smoking!

CHAPTER 28

Biventricular Devices

By placing a wire in both the left and right sides of the heart (the ventricles) and pacing both sides nearly simultaneously, doctors can improve the performance of the heart, including its ejection fraction. The biventricular approach can be used with a pacemaker or an ICD.

In patients with weak heart muscles and heart failure, these biventricular devices offer cardiac resynchronization therapy (CRT), which can help alleviate heart failure symptoms. Normally, the right and left heart chambers contract in synchrony to efficiently pump blood to the rest of the body. Patients with heart failure often have hearts that are out of synchrony, or dyssynchronous, meaning that left and right ventricles contract out of sequence, with a less effective pumping mechanism and resulting fluid buildup. Cardiac resynchronization therapy may restore synchrony by allowing the right and left sides of the heart to pump together more efficiently.

Certain criteria must be present for a person to qualify for this type of device (see table 28.1). These criteria include significant congestive heart failure (moderate to severe congestive heart failure, described as New York Heart Association class III or IV, despite treatment with optimal medical therapy), a low ejection fraction (35 percent or less), and the presence of a wide QRS complex on the ECG (see chapter 14), such as that which is caused by a bundle branch block. More recently, the results of the MADIT-CRT study

TABLE 28.1 *When do you need a biventricular device?*

- If you have moderate to severe heart failure despite being on optimal medical therapy, an EF of less than or equal to 35 percent, and a wide QRS duration on ECG
- If you have asymptomatic or mild heart failure with an EF of less than or equal to 30 percent with a wide QRS complex on ECG
- If you have low EF and are likely to need a lot of right ventricular pacing
- After an AV node ablation

were released. This study compared biventricular ICDs to regular ICDs in nearly two thousand patients asymptomatic or mildly symptomatic for heart failure (New York Heart Association class I and II) with an ejection fraction of 30 percent or less and a wide QRS complex. The results demonstrated a significant improvement in both survival and heart failure with a biventricular ICD.

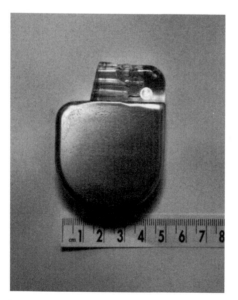

FIGURE 28.1. A biventricular implantable cardioverter defibrillator (ICD) pulse generator, used to treat people who have congestive heart failure and are at risk for sudden cardiac death.

Some physicians believe that biventricular pacing is helpful following ablation of the AV node in patients with drug-refractory atrial fibrillation. Physician judgment may also play a part in determining whether a biventricular device is needed. Appendix D provides a list of indications for a biventricular device, such as a pacemaker or ICD. Discuss your indication with your physician. (See also chapters 30, 31, and 32.)

Patients with a biventricular device should be taking routine heart failure medicines, such as diuretics, beta blockers, and an angiotensin-converting enzyme (ACE) inhibitor or an angiotensin II receptor blocker (ARB) or both.

A biventricular defibrillator (figure 28.1) uses an additional lead in the heart (referred to as the third lead). This additional lead is placed in the coronary sinus vein, which can pace the left ventricle. By pacing the left and right ventricle nearly simultaneously, pacemakers and ICDs improve heart function in approximately two out of three patients. The risks of this procedure are similar to those of other implantable devices. Although system problems are rare, patients should be aware that the more wires, leads, and parts involved, the greater the risk of system problems.

CHAPTER 29

Implantable Cardiac Monitors

Implantable cardiac monitors are useful in identifying very rare or infrequent abnormal cardiac rhythms that may result in light-headedness, dizziness, or loss of consciousness (see chapter 16). Implantable cardiac monitors are also called implantable loop recorders. They are the size of a small lighter. One such monitoring device may be seen in figure 29.1.

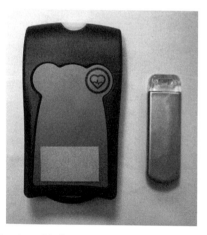

FIGURE 29.1. An implantable loop recorder (smaller device) and activator (larger device) used to monitor and record heart rhythms. The implantable loop recorder is implanted under the skin and can automatically record heart rhythm events. The activator can be used to trigger a heart rhythm recording when the person is experiencing symptoms such as palpitations, light-headedness, and dizziness.

An implantable cardiac monitor contains no wires (leads), can be implanted below the skin within minutes, and can remain implanted for up to three years. The purpose of the device is to monitor and record arrhythmias.

Information can be downloaded from the device, which can demonstrate significant rapid rhythms and slow rhythms that were previously undiagnosed despite a thorough work-up by a doctor. Many people who have received an implantable cardiac monitor have been discovered to have occult bradycardia, and these people benefited from a pacemaker implant. The risks of implanting a subcutaneous implantable cardiac monitor are mainly bleeding and infection. (See also chapters 30, 31, and 32.)

CHAPTER 30

Device Implant Procedures

If your cardiologist or electrophysiologist recommends a device implant to pace your heart or shock it back into a normal rhythm, you have almost certainly met guidelines established through careful analysis by physicians working collaboratively with the Heart Rhythm Society, the American College of Cardiology, and the American Heart Association. It is normal that a heart-related diagnosis and prescribed implant therapy will prompt concerns and questions from you and your family. This book was written in part to help you become more familiar with terminology, conditions, and treatment options, and to equip you with knowledgeable questions to ask your physician. This chapter discusses specific issues related to an implant procedure, but you should always feel free to ask your physician about your specific condition and how his or her recommendation for treatment compares to the guidelines established by the heart and heart rhythm–related societies.

Various implantable devices, placed for size comparison next to a standard pager, are pictured in figure 30.1. Even the largest devices, the biventricular ICDs on the top row, are smaller than the pager. While the devices continue to get both smaller and more advanced as technology improves, the implant procedure is still a surgical procedure, no matter how small the device.

There are at least five questions you should ask your doctor prior to your implant procedure (see table 30.1). Ask about the type of device you are receiving, and why this device. It is also ap-

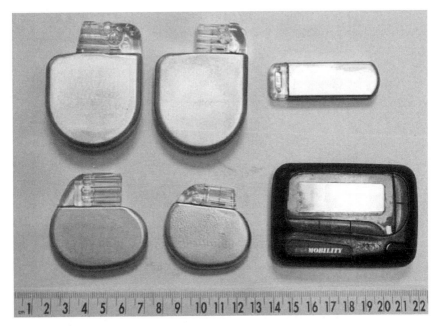

FIGURE 30.1. Various implantable devices in comparison to a standard pager. Two pacemakers are on the bottom row next to the pager. The largest implantable device, a biventricular ICD seen at top upper left, is still smaller than the pager. The implantable cardiac monitor, at top upper right, is the smallest device of them all.

propriate to find out the manufacturer of the device as well as the manufacturer's track record. Ask about the manufacturer's market share presence locally, nationally, and globally as well as about any recent recalls or safety advisories issued by the manufacturer or any other entity.

You and your family should ask about the experience the doctor has with these devices and what problems might be encountered during the procedure. That is, ask about the risks of the procedure. Find out how long the procedure will take, and request details about how it will be done. Also ask about any limitations you might experience after the procedure.

There are six things you should do after receiving a device

TABLE 30.1   *Five questions to ask your doctor before you get a device*

1. What type of device am I getting and why?
2. Who is the manufacturer and what is the company's track record?
3. How many of these devices have you put in and what problems have you seen?
4. What limitations will I have after the device? Can I drive? Can I have sex?
5. Is there any machinery I cannot operate?

TABLE 30.2   *Six things to do after you get a device*

1. Keep your wound clean and dry for one week following the implant.
2. Don't lift heavy items for 6 weeks.
3. Avoid MRIs unless you have received an MRI-compatible device (in which case, follow the specific instructions of your doctor).
4. Report any redness, swelling, or discharge from the wound. Follow up with your doctor within 2 weeks of the procedure.
5. Go for routine device checks with your doctor and see him or her personally at least once a year.
6. If you receive a device and are unsure of restrictions, the safest action is to call your doctor's office for instructions.

implant (table 30.2). You should keep your wound clean and dry for one week (most physicians recommend towel bathing for that week). After any implant in which a new lead is placed, patients are generally restricted from lifting heavy objects for at least 6 weeks. If your implantable device is not approved for MRI use, avoid MRI procedures; if you have received an MRI-compatible device, follow your doctor's specific instructions. Follow up with the doctor or his or her device-follow-up clinic within 2 weeks—or sooner if redness, swelling, or discharge from the surgical site occurs. The doctor should be notified immediately of other problems such as chest pain, light-headedness or dizziness, loss of consciousness, or frequent shocks.

Be vigilant about routine device checks either in person or via a remote monitoring service. Most implantable devices can now be monitored via the Internet, so physicians can routinely check on your condition and can immediately evaluate any specific symptoms through an Internet transmission. Yet even with remote monitoring, you should see your doctor in person at least once a year, or more often if necessary. Note that *remote monitoring services are not emergency services*, and you should understand how the remote monitoring is used by your doctor's office. Do not send a remote transmission from your device to your doctor's office without first contacting the office to verify that qualified personnel are on hand to receive it and interpret it. If not, you should seek medical attention in person if you have concerns.

Driving is generally not restricted unless you are still at significant risk for loss of consciousness (such as receiving an ICD after being revived from cardiac arrest), but you should always ask about specific instructions before returning to routines such as driving. Certain machinery and occupations may present some difficulties, and restrictions may be necessary if you work with radio waves, arc welding, strong magnetic fields, and other forms of electromagnetic interference. Pilots and drivers of public transportation must also discuss their particular situation and the necessity of a work restriction with their doctor. If you have any questions, or are experiencing any side effects or discomfort after your procedure, do not hesitate to contact your physician and to see him or her in person if necessary.

Common complications that may occur as the result of an implant, especially involving the placement of leads in the heart, are noted in table 30.3. In general, the larger and more complicated the system (and the more leads involved), the greater the risk for a complication or device failure. Biventricular ICDs have a higher complication rate than ICDs, which have higher risk than pacemakers. All devices have a risk for bleeding, infection, erosion through the skin, migration, malfunction, and even clot formation. Heart attack, stroke, and death are rare with any device but are more common in older people, people with more complicated medical conditions, and those who require more complicated procedures.

Implantable cardiac monitors and implantable loop recorders do not have leads and therefore do not carry the risk of perforation,

TABLE 30.3   *Complications and risks for any implantable device*

Infection	Lead dislodgement
Erosion (in which the device works its way out and "erodes" through the skin)	Device migration
	Device malfunction
	Damage to the heart, blood vessels, or other organs
Bleeding	
Collapse of the lung	Heart attack
Clot formation	Stroke
Perforation	Death

lung collapse, lead dislodgement, or damage to the heart and blood vessels. Other devices may carry these risks, including the risk of lung collapse if your doctor uses a needle to access a blood vessel near the lung. Again, these complications are experienced by a small minority of patients.

This book provides you and your family with the generally acceptable guidelines for device implants. Once you are comfortable with the fact that you meet these guidelines, you will, I hope, feel reassured that your physician is proceeding in your best interest, and you will understand that the benefits in this circumstance typically outweigh the risks. If you have any questions about whether a device is right for you, please discuss your concerns in advance with your doctor.

CHAPTER 31

Device Replacement and Lead Extraction

·····

As manufacturers continue to develop pacemakers and defibrillators, the devices tend to become smaller and more refined. A typical pacemaker lasts approximately eight years, and an ICD lasts approximately six years, depending on how often the devices are used. Eventually the device will need to be replaced simply because it has worn out. The procedure for replacement is similar to the procedure for the first implant (see previous chapters). Occasionally, people with implantable devices such as pacemakers, defibrillators, and biventricular devices develop complications such as a device-related infection or a lead malfunction. When a device-related infection occurs, it is important to extract all implantable material, including the leads and pulse generator. When a lead has malfunctioned, it may be important to replace it. A lead extraction may be advised when there are many leads in one blood vessel and no other site is available to place new leads. If a blood vessel is occluded, the occlusion may prevent the insertion of a new lead on the side where other leads and the device are functioning appropriately. By extracting the malfunctioning lead while maintaining access into the heart, a new lead can then be easily inserted. Common reasons for undergoing a lead extraction procedure are detailed in table 31.1.

When a lead is first implanted, it is either fastened to the heart by a screw at the end of the lead or by a tiny barb that can wedge into heart tissue. Eventually, over time, the lead is fused to the heart by tissue, which grows over the lead. Leads that have been

TABLE 31.1   *Three common reasons to undergo a lead extraction*

1. Device-related infection
2. Significant lead malfunction
3. Upgrading a device to a more complex system in which a lead or leads need to be added and an obstruction is found in the blood vessel, or many leads are already present in that blood vessel

implanted for more than one year are often difficult to remove, and special tools may be required to extract the leads, to avoid having it come apart within the body. Special expandable wires can be placed within the hollow lumen in the middle of the lead to firmly secure it in place from top to bottom. In addition, specially designed hollow tubes (or sheaths) are used to cut through the scar tissue that surrounds the lead and fuses it to the heart and blood vessels. These cutting sheaths can use laser or radiofrequency energy to cut through this scarring and free up the lead or leads for removal. The sheath can also provide an easy conduit for delivering new leads.

This technique of lead extraction is not without risks, including vessel and heart perforation and rupture with associated bleeding, and death. It is standard to have a cardiac surgeon immediately available should there be a need during such a procedure. Studies have shown that the more experience your doctor and your doctor's center has had with the procedure, the better the outcome. Ask your doctor about his or her personal experience, including the number of procedures performed as well as the results achieved.

CHAPTER 32

Recalls

In the United States, medical devices are regulated by the Food and Drug Administration (FDA). Before implantable devices are approved for use in patients, they must be thoroughly and rigorously tested by the manufacturer, and they must receive approval from the FDA. Implantable pacemakers, ICDs, and other devices are typically well-made, reliable machines, but they are not perfect. Each system is complex and has multiple components, including the case, battery, circuitry, capacitors, connectors, and leads. Occasionally, a malfunction may occur in one of the components. Very rarely, this malfunction may prevent the device from performing its life-saving function.

When an isolated defect randomly occurs in one of the device components, this event is called an isolated component failure. If the defect is in a noncritical area, it may be monitored and followed. When it disturbs the critical function of a device in a patient who is dependent on that function, the patient may collapse and even die. The term *pacemaker dependent* is used when a patient is completely dependent on the pacing function from the device and has little or no underlying heart rhythm. In this circumstance, if the pacemaker fails to put out any electrical pacing signal, the patient will likely collapse and potentially die.

When defects are not isolated and appear in a pattern that can be linked to a certain process, a larger scale problem may be involved. Patterns of device failure can be identified by doctors, manufacturers, and regulatory agencies. When a problem is not serious and has minimal impact on patient care, a safety advisory may be issued. Sometimes, a recall status may also be issued, depending on the severity of the problem. Recalls for devices and leads have been discussed in the news, and malpractice attorneys have contacted people who may have such devices to consider filing class action lawsuits. The reality is that even with many of the more publicized recalls, very few patients have died relative to the number of patients who have the recalled device or lead.

The FDA issues three classifications of recall (see table 32.1). The most serious classification is a class I recall, in which the device problem may severely impair the safety of the patient and has the potential for severe injury, including death. A class II recall might also have a risk for injury and death, but these outcomes are much less likely to occur. A class III recall is for a problem not likely to harm the patient, though there is a very remote chance of injury. The lower the classification number of the recall, the more likely the need for device intervention, such as device reprogramming, increased follow-up, or surgical revision or replacement.

When a recall is issued, the patient may be contacted by the manufacturer of their device by letter. The patient's doctor may also contact the patient by letter or by phone. If you are contacted about a device recall, try not to panic. Meet with your doctor and discuss the problem and what it may mean. Often, nothing needs to be done. Occasionally, devices may be reprogrammed, and sometimes patients might be followed more closely. Remote monitoring systems might help with follow-up, and programmed alarms or alerts may also help with identifying a malfunction before it is evident to the patient. Do not hesitate to discuss any issue with your doctor or the manufacturer.

TABLE 32.1   *Implantable device recall classification*

Recall class	Risk of injury and death	Likelihood of intervention
I	Highest	Highest
II	Intermediate	Intermediate
III	Lowest	Lowest

PART EIGHT

The Diseased Heart

CHAPTER 33

Heart Failure

···

Heart failure occurs when the heart weakens and cannot effectively pump blood to the rest of the body. Blood may back up from the left side of the heart into the lungs, causing congestion and shortness of breath. This is called *left heart failure*. Or blood may back up on the right side of the heart, resulting in leg swelling and swelling of other tissues and organs. This is called *right heart failure*. A person may have either right or left heart failure, or both.

Another classification of heart failure is related either to an impaired ability of the heart to pump blood (systolic dysfunction) or to an increased stiffness of the ventricles, which impairs blood filling (diastolic dysfunction). In heart failure, the heart's contraction, relaxation, or both may be affected. The primary differences between systolic heart failure and diastolic heart failure are shown in table 33.1.

Remodeling is a process in which the heart actually reshapes itself due to some injury or insult, such as long-standing fluid accumulation in the heart, which causes the heart muscle to stretch until it can no longer pump efficiently. Heart failure and many other cardiac disorders can cause remodeling.

In long-standing (or chronic) heart failure, many of the heart's repair mechanisms, which were initially compensating and allowing the heart to pump effectively, turn maladaptive and actually make the situation worse. When your heart is not ejecting enough blood to support the rest of your body, your body feels as though it is

TABLE 33.1 *Differences between systolic heart failure and diastolic heart failure*

Systolic heart failure	Diastolic heart failure
More common	Less common
Muscle weak or enlarged	Muscle thick or stiff
Impaired heart contraction	Impaired heart filling

under attack, and defense mechanisms come into play. The body has "feelers" outside the heart that determine whether these areas are getting enough blood. If these feelers realize the blood supply is low, they command blood vessels to become smaller and narrower. Think of a garden hose. When it is wide open, the water flows out smoothly. When you crimp the hose, it doesn't allow all the water to flow out. When the vessels clamp down, a strain is placed on the heart, causing fluid to be retained and preventing the heart from emptying. The result is an increase in symptoms such as shortness of breath.

Symptoms of heart failure have been classified by the New York Heart Association into four classes (table 33.2). Patients who are class I are essentially without symptoms and have no limitations on activity. Patients with class II congestive heart failure have mild symptoms that occur only with a great degree of exertion. Class III patients have marked limitation of activity, and symptoms occur upon mild exertion. Class IV patients are symptomatic at rest. The symptoms of heart failure include shortness of breath, leg swelling,

TABLE 33.2 *The New York Heart Association classification of congestive heart failure*

Class I: Patients with no limitation of activities; they suffer no symptoms from ordinary activities.

Class II: Patients with a slight limitation of activity; they are comfortable at rest and with mild exertion.

Class III: Patients with marked limitation of activity; they are comfortable only at rest.

Class IV: Patients are symptomatic even at rest, and physical activity brings on discomfort.

decreased exercise tolerance, fatigue, and light-headedness or dizziness and confusion (table 33.3). Causes of congestive heart failure include anything that results in heart disease (table 33.4), such as ischemia or lack of blood flow to the heart, a heart attack, a weak or thickened heart muscle, leaky or tight heart valves, inherited conditions, viral infections, and drug toxicities, including alcohol abuse.

If your doctor is concerned about the possibility of heart failure, he or she may order a number of diagnostic tests, such as an echocardiogram, a noninvasive stress test, an angiogram, and a chest x-ray. Lab tests may include blood chemistries, complete blood counts, and levels of electrolytes, liver enzymes, BNP (B-type natriuretic peptides), and homocysteine.

The best treatment for heart failure includes moderate exercise and a healthy diet. Your doctor may prescribe medications such as a beta blocker, an aldosterone inhibitor, an angiotensin-converting enzyme (ACE) inhibitor, an angiotensin II receptor blocker (ARB),

TABLE 33.3   *Symptoms of heart failure*

Shortness of breath	Confusion
Leg swelling	Coughing or wheezing
Decreased exercise tolerance	Weight gain
Fatigue	Palpitations
Light-headedness, dizziness	

TABLE 33.4   *Causes of heart failure*

Lack of blood flow to the heart (ischemia)
Presence of a heart attack (myocardial infarction)
Weak heart muscle (cardiomyopathy)
Thickened heart muscle (such as occurs with hypertrophic cardiomyopathy)
Leaky heart valves (valvular regurgitation)
Tight heart valves (stenosis)
Inherited conditions
Drug toxicity
Heart rhythm problems (arrhythmias) that weaken the heart muscle
   (tachycardia-induced cardiomyopathy)
Infection (such as a virus)

diuretics, and possibly digitalis (see chapter 25). People who have heart failure are at risk for sudden cardiac arrest caused by ventricular tachycardia or ventricular fibrillation. ICDs have been demonstrated to prolong life in people who have heart failure. Devices that can pace both the left and right ventricles are called *biventricular devices*; they can improve heart function beyond what can be achieved with medications.

A person may qualify for a biventricular ICD if he or she has an EF of 35 percent or less, has symptomatic congestive heart failure (New York Heart Association class III or IV), is on optimal medical therapy, and has a wide QRS complex on ECG. Improvement in symptoms may be observed in about two of every three patients who have met the preceding criteria. More recently, the MADIT-CRT study demonstrated that biventricular ICDs improve survival with fewer heart failure interventions even in asymptomatic or mildly symptomatic heart failure patients (New York Heart Association class I or II) with an EF of 30 percent or less and a wide QRS complex. If you are experiencing symptoms of congestive heart failure or have a very weak heart as indicated by an EF of 30 percent or less, you may want to discuss the option of a biventricular device with your doctor (see chapter 28).

CHAPTER 34

Cardiomyopathy

....

The heart is composed of muscle cells. In a normal heart, all the cells in the heart work together to complete their tasks, which, combined, allow the heart to pump effectively. When the heart is diseased, however, it cannot accomplish its tasks efficiently. Cardiomyopathy is a weak or abnormal heart muscle: *cardio* (heart), *myo* (muscle), and *pathy* (disease process) = heart muscle disease.

Cardiomyopathy may be debilitating. There are three main types: dilated, hypertrophic, and restrictive. This chapter discusses the different types of cardiomyopathy, their causes, and the possible treatments.

People with cardiomyopathies may be symptom-free or highly symptomatic. Symptoms differ from one person to the next. The most common are those of heart failure, including shortness of breath and leg swelling. People who have a cardiomyopathy may experience periods of dizziness or syncope (passing out). They may appear pale, and they may have chest pain. Many people with cardiomyopathy are at risk for abnormal heart rhythms (arrhythmias), particularly ventricular arrhythmias. Medical and device therapy are often prescribed based on the patient's ejection fraction and any heart failure symptoms.

Dilated Cardiomyopathy

Dilated cardiomyopathy is a common cause of heart failure. The heart muscle enlarges, and the muscle walls become thin. There are many causes of dilated cardiomyopathy:

ischemic
idiopathic
hypertensive
valvular
chemotherapy/radiation induced
peripartum (induced by pregnancy)
alcohol related
inherited

Ischemic cardiomyopathy is the most common form of dilated cardiomyopathy. It is the direct result of coronary artery disease. The term *ischemic* refers to the heart being deprived of oxygen from impaired coronary artery circulation, impairing the heart's ability to contract. Chapter 12 discusses the process of atherosclerosis (hardening of the arteries) and its linkage to sudden cardiac arrest. Acutely, plaque can rupture within a coronary artery, depriving a specific region of the heart of oxygen. An abrupt coronary artery blockage may cause death of heart muscle tissue (also called a heart attack, or myocardial infarction). The scar from a heart attack may also provide the necessary substrate for ventricular tachycardia or ventricular fibrillation. Although I am discussing ischemic cardiomyopathy under the category of dilated cardiomyopathy, it is possible that the heart itself may not dilate, even though there is a focal area of scar from a prior heart attack. In many people, however, the heart muscle thins and eventually dilates.

Many people with coronary artery disease are treated with heart medications, which are discussed in chapter 25. Chapters 12, 15, 18, and 19 discuss imaging and treatment modalities, including percutaneous coronary intervention and stenting. Some people need coronary artery bypass surgery to achieve complete revascularization. Through primary prevention, the ICD has been demonstrated to improve survival in patients with a history of prior myocardial infarction and an EF of 30 percent or less. Many studies have also demonstrated the utility of this device in the secondary prevention of sudden cardiac arrest in people with ischemic cardiomyopathies.

Idiopathic dilated cardiomyopathy is another common form of dilated cardiomyopathy. The term is used when the etiology is unknown. Causes may come from a variety of sources, including an unknown genetic cause or infection.

Cardiomyopathy may result from long-standing high blood pressure (hypertension). Initially the heart muscle may thicken as a result of the high blood pressure. Later, the heart muscle may give way and dilate.

Disease of the heart valves (also called *valvular disease*) occurs as a result of a leaky or tight mitral or aortic valve. Both of these valves are located on the left side of the heart (see chapter 1). The mitral valve separates the left atrium (top chamber) from the left ventricle (bottom chamber), and the aortic valve is the valve that controls the outflow of oxygen-rich blood that leaves the left ventricle through the aorta and is distributed to the rest of the body. If there is backflow of blood, valvular cardiomyopathy may result. When heart valves leak, the chambers (atria and ventricles) do not empty completely, the heart muscle may stretch, and over time, the heart muscle may weaken and the chambers may dilate. When valve disease is severe or when symptoms occur, valve repair or replacement surgery may be necessary.

Chemotherapeutic agents and radiation used in some cancer treatments may cause dilated cardiomyopathy. A cardiac work-up is recommended for most people before they receive certain chemotherapeutic agents. People with underlying cardiac disease are at greater risk for developing this type of cardiomyopathy.

Pregnant women or women who have given birth within the previous six months are at risk for developing peripartum dilated cardiomyopathy. This type is usually limited and resolves on its own. Alcohol abuse, a toxin to the heart, may cause a dilated cardiomyopathy. Binge drinking can bring on heart rhythm problems (called *holiday heart*).

Other inflammatory causes and known infections can also weaken the heart muscle. Direct inflammation of the heart muscle is called *myocarditis*. Noninfectious causes of heart inflammation include those caused by autoimmune disorders such as systemic lupus erythematosus. In addition, myocarditis may be present in patients with peripartum dilated cardiomyopathy; however, heart inflammation is most often caused by a viral infection. Specific viruses, parasites, and bacteria may attack the heart muscle and weaken it. Myocarditis may arise from bacteria called *Borrelia burgdorferi*, found on a deer tick, as a result of a tick bite, as is seen in Lyme disease. Specific heart infections can be treated with antiviral or antibiotics depending on their specific cause. In other cases, there are no specific targeted treatments available other than supportive measures. In some instances, the effects from the infections are short lived and heart function improves. In others, the infection inflicts permanent damage on the heart, and medication plus device therapy should be considered. In severe cases, heart transplantation may be considered.

An inherited condition in which the right ventricle dilates as the result of fat deposited in the right ventricular muscle is called arrhythmogenic right ventricular dysplasia (see chapter 35). This dysplasia makes the person more likely to develop ventricular tachycardia, and an ICD may be required.

Cardiac transplantation is the last resort for patients with cardiomyopathies whose symptoms are not resolved from standard medical or surgical treatments. Treatments for different types of dilated cardiomyopathy are listed in table 34.1. In general, treatment is directed to the underlying cardiac condition, and device-based therapies such as ICDs are also considered when indicated. For example, in a person with a history of a heart attack and symptomatic ventricular tachycardia, the underlying condition (coronary artery disease) might require revascularization by PCI and stenting and medical treatment with acetylsalicylic acid, clopidogrel, statins, and

TABLE 34.1   *Dilated cardiomyopathy types and treatments*

Types	Treatments
Ischemic	ACE inhibitors, ARBs, beta blockers, device therapy, revascularization
Idiopathic	ACE inhibitors, ARBs, beta blockers, device therapy
Hypertensive	ACE inhibitors, ARBs, beta blockers, device therapy
Valvular	ACE inhibitors, ARBs, hydralazine/nitrates, valve surgery (repair or replacement), device therapy
Chemotherapeutic/ radiation induced	ACE inhibitors, ARBs, beta blockers, device therapy
Pregnancy-induced	ACE inhibitors, ARBs, beta blockers, device therapy if condition persists
Alcohol-related	ACE inhibitors, ARBs, beta blockers, abstinence from alcohol, device therapy
Inflammation- or infection-induced	ACE inhibitors, ARBs, beta blockers, device therapy, treatment of specific cause
Inherited (arrhythmo-genic right ventricular dysplasia)	ACE inhibitors, ARBs, beta blockers, sotalol, device therapy

a beta blocker. If the EF is decreased (less than 50 percent) or the patient has congestive heart failure, the patient should receive additional medical treatment with an ACE inhibitor, an ARB, or both. An ICD would be recommended to treat any recurrent episodes of ventricular tachycardia.

Hypertrophic Cardiomyopathy

Hypertrophic cardiomyopathy (HCM) is a condition typically characterized by a thickened heart muscle. Hypertrophic means "enlargement." In this disease, the heart's cells are enlarged, which makes the walls of the heart thicker in diameter. Think of a thin rubber band that can be easily stretched (just as the heart can easily stretch), and then think of a thicker rubber band. You can feel the increased tension when you try to stretch the thicker rubber band.

More than half of HCM cases are caused by genetic mutations. (A good resource for researching genetic disorders is the National Institutes of Health.) Another cause for this type of cardiomyopathy is long-standing high blood pressure, which may also cause heart wall muscles to thicken. Hypertrophic cardiomyopathy may be associated with an obstruction that blocks blood from leaving the heart, called *hypertrophic obstructive cardiomyopathy*.

A thickened muscle in and of itself makes it more likely that a person will have ventricular tachycardia or ventricular fibrillation, and hypertrophic cardiomyopathy is best treated with an ICD. Diagnostic evaluations usually include an ECG and echocardiography. The ECG is not considered diagnostic, but it may assist in the diagnosis, while the echocardiogram will give pictures to demonstrate the degree of wall thickness. Genetic testing is available for those suspected of having a genetic component (see chapter 35 for a discussion of hereditary conditions).

Treatment usually relates to the symptoms. Drug therapies may include beta blockers and calcium channel blockers. Amiodarone may be useful for treating persistent abnormal heart rhythms such as atrial fibrillation. It may also be useful in suppressing recurrent ventricular tachycardia in patients with an ICD. Interventions may include a surgical procedure to remove part of the heart muscle (septal myotomy-myomectomy), or a catheterization procedure in which alcohol is delivered down a coronary artery to injure the middle of the heart and improve overall function (alcohol septal ablation procedure). ICDs are usually recommended for patients who are symptomatic or who are at risk for arrhythmias. Eventually, genetic medical therapies (which are currently investigational) may have a role in the treatment of this disorder.

HCM is the leading cause of sudden death in athletes younger than 35 years old.

Restrictive Cardiomyopathy

A restrictive cardiomyopathy occurs when the ventricles are non-compliant and cannot fill properly during the resting phase (diastole) of the heart cycle. The most common cause is a disease called *cardiac amyloidosis*, in which an abnormal protein builds up in the muscle. Amyloid protein buildup can occur in any organ in the body, not just the heart. Diagnosis is usually made by echocardiogram and a heart or tissue biopsy, which helps to confirm the diagnosis.

Other causes of restrictive cardiomyopathy include idiopathic causes, malignancy, radiation therapy, heart transplantation, and other infiltrative disorders, such as hemochromatosis (iron deposition in the heart).

Treatment includes such medications as nitrates, beta blockers, and calcium channel blockers. Patients are advised to avoid products containing salt (sodium) and to carefully manage their weight. Diuretics may worsen symptoms and should be used with caution. An ICD may be useful to treat patients at risk for ventricular tachycardia or ventricular fibrillation.

CHAPTER 35

Hereditary Conditions

Each cell in your body contains genes, which are the body's blueprints for development, growth, and functioning. Located within these genes are proteins called *deoxyribonucleic acid* (DNA). Genes are programmed before birth to provide our cells and to tell the organs of our body to perform specific tasks. Let's say a gene is named H-E-A-R-T, and its programmed function is to pump blood throughout the body. If that same gene is misspelled, say E-H-A-R-T, the programmed function would change, just as if you were reading the word E-H-A-R-T and did not recognize it to mean "heart." In this way, how genes are spelled (or coded) gives meaning to their function.

One major function of the heart is to support a normal heart rhythm. If the function (the spelling of the code) is altered, arrhythmias can arise. One major problem with these hereditary cardiac disorders is the risk for ventricular arrhythmias and sudden cardiac arrest. Tragically, some patients who possess genetic disorders are not identified (unless a strong family history is present) until they experience sudden cardiac death.

With many genetic disorders, it is necessary for only one parent (not both parents) to have the gene in order to pass it on to the child. It is now known that most diseases have a genetic basis that may or may not be passed from parent to child. For the purpose of this section, the focus is on genetic diseases related to heart rhythm problems that *can* be passed this way. Evidence suggests that our environment can affect how these genetic disorders express themselves. Genetic defects discussed in this chapter are arrhythmogenic right ventricular dysplasia, hypertrophic cardiomyopathy (see chapter 34), long QT syndrome, and Brugada syndrome. See table 35.1 for a list of the common gene subtypes of these disorders. Later in this chapter, I discuss genetic testing as well as the treatment for people with hereditary cardiac disorders.

Arrhythmogenic Right Ventricular Dysplasia

Arrhythmogenic right ventricular dysplasia is a heart disorder typically seen in young adults. It is associated with abnormal heart rhythms. In this disorder, fat deposits in the heart muscle make these patients, especially young individuals or athletes, more likely to develop ventricular arrhythmias and possibly suffer sudden cardiac death. The disorder may be identified through ventricular tachycardia, abnormal echocardiogram, and cardiac MRI (which may demonstrate fat deposits in the right ventricular wall). Treatments include lifestyle changes, antiarrhythmic medications, and an ICD.

TABLE 35.1   *Common associated gene subtypes for inherited rhythm disorders*

Disorder	Gene subtypes
Arrhythmogenic right ventricular dysplasia (fat deposits in right ventricular wall)	PKP2, DSP, GSG2
Hypertrophic cardiomyopathy (thickened heart muscle)	MYH7, MYBPC3
Long QT syndrome (has specific ECG pattern)	KCNQ1 (long QT1); KCNH2 (long QT2); SCN5A (long QT3)
Brugada syndrome (has specific ECG pattern)	SCN5A

Source: T. J. Cohen, *Practical Electrophysiology,* 2nd ed. (Malvern, PA: HMP Communications, 2009), p. 190.

Hypertrophic Cardiomyopathy

Numerous genes have been implicated in causing hypertrophic cardiomyopathy, which may cause thickening of the heart muscle. See chapter 34 for a discussion of this condition.

Long QT Syndrome

The first family identified as having long QT (LQT) syndrome was reported in 1957. This disorder was originally called Romano-Ward syndrome, though that term is outdated. Research has since demonstrated that many different genetic defects cause long QT syndrome; in fact, scientists have identified more than 300 mutations on many different genes. With this knowledge, long QT syndrome has subsequently been divided into numbered categories (LQTS1, LQTS2, LQTS3, and so on).

The most common type of LQT syndrome is type 2, which was identified in 1994. The disorder is demonstrated by a prolongation of the QT segment on the ECG. On a routine ECG, this QT change may not always be apparent. Your doctor may send you for exercise tests to elicit changes in the QT interval that would raise suspicion of this disorder. Treatment may include medications such as beta blockers, environmental restrictions such as a modified exercise regimen and avoidance of noise or startling events, and possibly even an ICD. The latter device-based treatment should be considered for people with serious symptoms that cannot be controlled by medications and lifestyle modifications. Please note that there are many drugs you should avoid if you have LQT syndrome (table 35.2). These drugs have a tendency to lengthen the QT interval. They include diuretics (which can cause electrolyte abnormalities that can lengthen the QT interval), stimulants of any kind, and certain "anti" drugs such as antibiotics, antidepressants, antihistamines, anticonvulsants, and antiarrhythmics. Please note that this list is not exhaustive; you may want to consult the following resources—Heart Rhythm Society, "Long QT Syndrome," www

TABLE 35.2   *Some drugs to avoid in long QT syndrome*

"Anti" drugs (*see also* "Psychiatric medications" below)
    Antiarrhythmics
        ibutilide
        procainamide
        quinidine
        disopyramide
        sotalol
        dofetilide
        propafenone
    Antibiotics
        macrolides such as erythromycin
        fluoroquinolones
    Anticonvulsants
    Antihistamines
    Antihypertensives
Diuretics (can lower electrolytes such as potassium and lengthen QT interval)
Gastrointestinal motility drugs
Migraine medications
Psychiatric medications
    stimulants such as methylphenidate
    antidepressants such as tricyclic antidepressants and SSRIs
    antipsychotics such as haloperidol
    tranquilizers

.hrspatients.org/patients/heart_disorders/long_qt_syndrome.asp; and Care, "Medications to Avoid," www.longqt.org/medications .html—and consult with your doctor.

Brugada Syndrome

Brugada syndrome is an inherited condition placing the patient at risk of sudden death. In the 1980s, the Centers for Disease Control reported a high incidence of sudden death in young Asian immigrants from Thailand. In Thailand the disorder was known as LaiTai (death during sleep). In 1992, the Brugada brothers identified the disease now known as Brugada syndrome. Genetic investigation led researchers to identify the culprit as a defective gene affecting specialized channels within heart cells. On ECG, a specialized pattern of Brugada waves may be noted, which appear as concave upward ST segments. Sudden death in this condition is usually caused by ventricular fibrillation. The condition is best treated with an ICD.

Diagnostic Tests for Hereditary Disorders

Tests that may be ordered in the diagnosis of these conditions and disorders include the following:

a twelve-lead ECG
a special computerized ECG called *signal-averaged ECG* (SAECG)
echocardiography
cardiac MRI
Holter monitoring
exercise stress testing
electrophysiology testing
coronary angiography (cardiac catheterization)

Certain blood tests can identify the genes responsible for inherited conditions. These tests have been expensive and have sometimes not been covered by routine health insurance. As the tests are more commonly practiced and more readily available, the costs have started to decrease and some insurance companies and government-sponsored health plans are offering reimbursement. An important step in expanding genetic testing occurred on May 21, 2008, when President George W. Bush signed the Genetic Information Nondiscrimination Act (GINA). This law prohibits discrimination on the basis of information obtained through genetic testing as it relates to employment and insurance coverage.

Since its inception, genetic testing has raised ethical issues for some people. Whether patients are tested with traditional diagnostic tools or with genetic testing, they need to be aware of the implications to other family members when one person is identified as having a genetic disorder. Some patients do not want others to know about their condition, and some individuals do not want to deal with the psychological effects of knowing they have a life-threatening condition. Generally, however, identifying the risk factors through diagnostic or genetic testing is important to patients and other family members so that they can be properly treated with drug or other medical therapies. Unfortunately, many families only learn about genetic testing after the tragedy of sudden cardiac death strikes a parent or child. Now that privacy of genetic testing is protected and discrimination is prohibited through federal law, there is more reason than ever for patients to fully discuss the option of genetic testing with their physician if there is a family history or suspected history of these hereditary conditions.

Make your physician aware of a strong family history of passing out (syncope), with or without sudden death. If a close family member has died suddenly, even if it was a parent or grandparent and it occurred twenty years ago, share that information with your physician. If a family is identified as being at risk for sudden cardiac death, your doctor can increase surveillance of all family members, which will make appropriate and timely treatment options more likely.

Treatment Options for People with Hereditary Cardiac Disorders

The goal for individuals who are identified with hereditary disorders is prevention of sudden cardiac death. Treatment may include lifestyle modifications (avoiding strenuous exercise, avoiding caffeine and cigarettes, limiting alcohol intake), medications (beta blockers are helpful in treating long QT syndrome), ablation therapies, and possibly implantation of an ICD. Treatment in the future may include genetic therapies, such as the delivery of engineered genes into a patient's cells to treat the specific genetic defect.

My family consisted of my mother, father, and three children (including myself). In the early 1970s, my mother experienced an unexplained syncopal event. Some six or seven years later, my brother, then 15 years old, had a similar fainting spell and was in a semicomatose state for about 24 hours. During his subsequent hospitalization, various tests were conducted, and doctors concluded that he might have had a drug overdose or drug reaction. To this day, my family does not understand why doctors would have made such a diagnosis, since they never identified a drug in his system that may have caused the event.

Several years later, while on vacation, my brother collapsed again. Friends administered CPR, and he was taken to a local hospital. When he was well enough to return home, my parents took him to a local cardiologist, who referred him to a well-known university hospital several hours away. Physicians and researchers there were doing extensive work on arrhythmias and had identified the patterns and traits of long QT syndrome, which can result in arrhythmias, syncope, and even sudden death. An extensive cardiology exam identified my brother as having long QT. At their recommendation, my family was given ECGs, and my mother's ECG also showed the patterns of the condition (essentially an elongated pause at the end of the heartbeat). Both my mother and my brother were put on beta blocker therapy. No other family members were identified as having the condition. During this time, my family agreed to participate in a clinical research project, which eventually led to the first identification of genetic markers for long QT as well as the first commercial genetic tests for patients. Some twelve years later, I was married and had children. While my ECG had shown no trait of long QT, I routinely took my young children for an ECG, given the family history. At the age of 5, my eldest daughter's ECG showed the traits. While genetic tests for long QT were not widely available and were not covered by insurance, my children and I were genetically tested. All three of us were identified as carriers of one of the genetic abnormalities associated with long QT.

We are all on beta blocker therapy and have shown no symptoms, but every year we consult with an electrophysiologist, who monitors our heart health. The kids are now teenagers, and as a precaution, they do not play competitive sports, but they dance, play tennis, and are otherwise normal and active. My family has donated and advocated for the placement of automatic external defibrillators (AEDs) in our children's schools. My younger brother, who was the source of the original diagnosis, has had an implantable cardioverter defibrillator for more than fifteen years because of chronic issues related to his condition.

While not happy with the diagnosis, I am certainly thankful that my wife and I took the family history seriously and consulted with medical experts to get the appropriate care. My wife and I also make sure that the physicians we see for other health issues understand the condition and do not prescribe drugs that can trigger arrhythmias. Finally, we work very hard to make sure that our children learn to take responsibility for their condition. Just like people with diabetes must watch what they eat and take insulin, our kids understand the importance of watching their diet, sticking to a regular exercise routine, and taking their medicine on time.

PART NINE

Prevention and Resuscitation

CHAPTER 36

Preventing Heart Disease

To prevent heart disease, it is important for you to eat a healthy diet, exercise in moderation, and work with your doctor to identify known risks for heart disease and treat them accordingly. A prudent diet is one that is recommended by the American Heart Association and is low in saturated fats. This kind of diet will help to maintain a healthy weight and body mass index (BMI). BMI is a measure of body fat based on height and weight (see table 36.1). To find out more information on BMI and to calculate your own BMI, visit the National Institutes of Health Web site at www.nhlbi.nih.gov/health/public/heart/obesity/wecan/learn-it/bmi-chart.htm. In addition to consuming a diet low in saturated fat, individuals with high blood pressure should limit salt intake and integrate regular exercise into their routine—such as walking for 30 minutes three or four times a week. These steps can be helpful in lowering your risk for heart disease.

Certain risk factors may predispose an individual to heart disease. These include cigarette smoking, high blood pressure, high cholesterol, diabetes, and a family history of heart disease. The first four risk factors may be reduced by appropriate medication and diet. The final risk factor will require additional vigilance and care by you, together with the help of your doctor.

If your father or brother had a heart attack before age 55, or if your mother or sister had one before age 65, you are at a higher risk for a heart attack. Women should be aware that after menopause,

TABLE 36.1   *Body mass index (BMI) categories*

BMI (kg/m²)	Category
Less than 18.5	Underweight
18.5 to 24.9	Normal weight
25 to 29.9	Overweight
Greater than 30	Obese

You can calculate your BMI as follows:
Using the metric system: BMI (kg/m²) = weight in kilograms ÷ (height in meters)².
Using the English system: BMI (kg/m²) = weight in pounds × 703 ÷ (height in inches)².

TABLE 36.2   *Modifiable and nonmodifiable risk factors*

Modifiable risk factors	Nonmodifiable risk factors
Smoking: Quit smoking.	Age: Incidence of heart disease rises with age (55 years or older for women).
High cholesterol: Avoid fatty foods and excessive alcohol, exercise regularly, consider cholesterol-lowering drugs.	Gender: Heart disease is more common in men than in women, but both sexes have an equal chance of developing heart disease after age 60.
Diabetes mellitus: Treat with diet and medications.	
Obesity: Avoid overeating, consume a healthy diet, and exercise to maintain appropriate body mass index (BMI).	Family history: The chance of disease increases with the number of family members who suffer from heart disease.
Stress: Relax, using relaxation techniques if necessary.	

they are equally at risk as men for heart disease. Being aware of your personal risks for heart disease and taking proper action to help reduce these risks is an important step in preventing heart disease. Modifiable and nonmodifiable risk factors for cardiac disease are described in table 36.2.

CHAPTER 37

Cardiopulmonary Resuscitation (CPR)

....

Cardiopulmonary resuscitation (CPR) is a method of resuscitating an unconscious person who has no significant blood pressure or who has inadequate circulation by providing chest compressions and ventilation (breaths delivered to the person's airway). By definition, a person who does not have a palpable pulse has inadequate circulation. When someone collapses from any cause and is not breathing and has no palpable pulse, CPR must be initiated *immediately* and *effectively* if the person is going to have any chance for survival. By alternately compressing the chest over the lower part of the person's chest bone (called the *sternum*) and then allowing it to relax, it is possible to help circulate blood throughout the body. In addition, by providing mouth to mouth ventilation to the person, you support the breathing, or pulmonary, component of *cardiopulmonary* resuscitation. In general, thirty chest compressions are given, followed by two breaths, until a defibrillator arrives at the scene.

Most cases of sudden cardiac arrest are caused by ventricular tachycardia or ventricular fibrillation, which almost always requires prompt defibrillation to achieve a good outcome and a successful resuscitation. CPR courses are available through local hospitals, support groups such as the Sudden Cardiac Arrest Association, and organizations such as the American Heart Association and the American Red Cross. These courses will teach the ABCs of CPR, which are *Airway access*, *Breathing*, and *Circulation*. A CPR certification card is given to participants when they complete the course.

The steps in performing CPR on an unconscious person are detailed in figure 37.1. The first step is to assess the person and make sure that he or she is unconscious and unresponsive. If you think this is an emergency, it is imperative to call 911 and immediately assess the airway, breathing, and circulation. The airway can be assessed by listening and feeling for breathing from the person's nose and mouth. Also, look to see if the chest is rising and falling from respiration. If the person is not breathing and there is no airway obstruction, then two breaths should be given.

Check the person's pulse, either at the neck level, where the

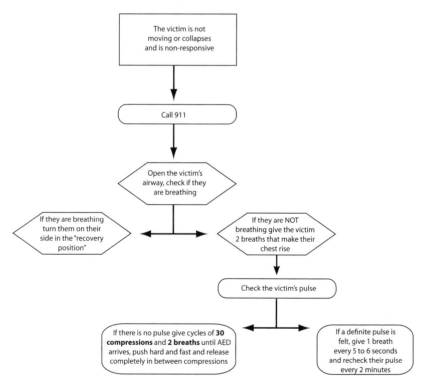

FIGURE 37.1. The proper protocol when dealing with an unconscious person and the initiation of CPR.

carotid pulsation can be felt, or at the wrist, where the radial pulse may be felt. If there is no pulse, initiate CPR: thirty chest compressions followed by two breaths. If the pulse recovers and the person is still not breathing, give one breath every 5 to 6 seconds.

It is important to practice the techniques of CPR periodically

TABLE 37.1   *How CPR should be performed on adults, children, and infants*

First, call 911.

Maneuver	Adult (older than 8 years)	Child (1 to 8 years)	Infant (under 1 year)
How to open airway	Head tilt, chin lift	Head tilt, chin lift	Head tilt, chin lift
How often to breathe mouth to mouth	2 breaths at 2 seconds	2 breaths at 2 seconds (make chest rise)	Two breaths at 2 seconds (make chest rise)
Where to check pulse	Carotid (neck) or radial (wrist)	Brachial (arm) or femoral (groin)	Brachial (arm) or femoral (groin)
Where to do compressions	Lower half of sternum, between nipples	Lower half of sternum, between nipples	Just below nipple line
How to do compressions	Push hard and fast with heel of one hand with other hand on top	Push hard and fast with heel of one hand, possibly with second hand on top	Push hard and fast with two fingers
How deeply to compress	1.5 to 2 inches	Approx. ⅓ to ½ the depth of the chest	Approx. ⅓ to ½ the depth of the chest
How fast to compress	Approx. 100 compressions per minute	Approx. 100 compressions per minute	Approx. 100 compressions per minute

Source: Derived from 2005 American Heart Association "Guidelines for Cardiopulmonary Resuscitation and Emergency Cardiovascular Care," *Circulation* 112, supplement 1 (2005): IV-1-211.

to retain the appropriate skills. Recertification in CPR (basic life support) is required every two years to maintain certification. Important information about performing CPR on adults, children, and infants is provided in table 37.1.

The airway must be opened by tilting the head backwards and lifting the chin. Each breath should be given in pairs of two, each lasting 2 seconds in duration. Remember the numbers 30 and 2 for the number of chest compressions followed by breaths, then chest compression followed again by breaths, and so on. Chest compressions should be performed on the lower half of the chest bone (sternum) at a depth of 1.5 to 2 inches, with a rate of approximately 100 compressions per minute. Performing chest compressions to the rhythm of the refrain of the Bee Gees' song "Stayin' Alive" (from the movie *Saturday Night Fever*) is useful for approximating this rate. Remember: "Ah, ha, ha, ha, stayin' alive, stayin' alive" (repeat, repeat, repeat). The compressions are performed with the heel of one hand on the chest, and the other hand on top of that one.

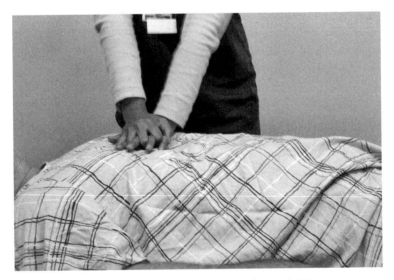

FIGURE 37.2. The compression phase, or active phase, of CPR. Compressions are administered over the chest bone.

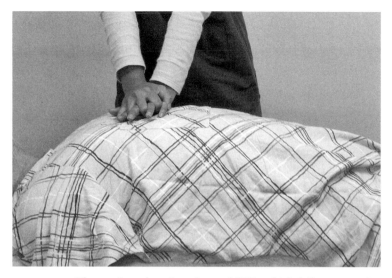

FIGURE 37.3. The passive relaxation phase of CPR, which follows an active compression administered to the chest.

Strong and effective chest compressions are essential to help provide oxygen and blood flow throughout the body.

How to perform appropriate CPR is demonstrated in figures 37.2 and 37.3. During chest compression (figure 37.2), air is pressed out of the lungs, and blood is expelled from the heart to the rest of the body. The passive relaxation phase of CPR (figure 37.3) follows the compression phase. During the passive relaxation phase, the chest passively expands, which helps the lungs to fill with air and the heart to fill with blood.

CHAPTER 38

Automatic External Defibrillator (AED)

An automatic external defibrillator (AED) is a simple self-guided electronic device, usually the size of a lunch box, that is used to shock a person out of ventricular tachycardia or ventricular fibrillation. Skin patches are connected to the chest and hooked into the AED (see figure 38.1). An illustration is typically provided in the AED kit to demonstrate where the patches should be placed on the chest. The AED orally guides you through the usage of the system, telling you how to detect the heart rhythm abnormality and how to deliver a shock.

AEDs are often successful in treating life-threatening arrhythmias like ventricular tachycardia and ventricular fibrillation. AEDs are available in many public areas such as airports, schools, supermarkets, and sports arenas. Figure 38.1 shows how an AED works.

Who Should Learn CPR and Learn How to Use an AED?

Anyone who is at risk for heart rhythm problems or sudden cardiac arrest, or who knows someone who is at risk for any of these problems, should learn CPR and how to use an AED. People overseeing large areas where people congregate, such as shopping malls, supermarkets, government centers, large businesses, arenas and stadiums, churches, temples, bus and train stations, airports, any other means of mass transportation, as well as at competitive sporting

How an AED Works

When someone collapses from sudden cardiac arrest, damage to the brain and vital organs begins in as little as four minutes if untreated. Often the heart does not stop completely, but goes into ventricular fibrillation, in which the heart quivers rapidly but does not pump blood effectively. A shock from an AED can reverse this condition, restore the heart's natural rhythm, and prevent permanent damage and death, but is much more effective if it is delivered in the first few minutes after collapse. It is important to perform CPR until the arrival of a defibrillator for use.

Using an AED is easy.
Just follow these simple steps:

1 Turn on the AED.

2 Attach the electrode pads to the victim's chest.

3 Press the ANALYZE button or allow the device to analyze automatically.

4 Press the SHOCK button if advised.

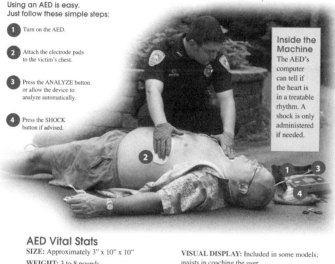

Inside the Machine
The AED's computer can tell if the heart is in a treatable rhythm. A shock is only administered if needed.

AED Vital Stats

SIZE: Approximately 3" x 10" x 10"

WEIGHT: 3 to 8 pounds

BATTERIES: Long-lasting lithium with no recharging required

VOICE PROMPTS: Included in all models (many with foreign language options), provide step-by-step instructions automatically when the unit is turned on

VISUAL DISPLAY: Included in some models; assists in coaching the user

LIST PRICE: About $1,300 to $2,000 for a single unit

For more information, please visit
www.suddencardiacarrest.org

FIGURE 38.1. "How an AED works." Reproduced with permission from the Sudden Cardiac Arrest Association.

events at any level should learn CPR and how to use an AED. A person surviving a sudden cardiac arrest in the community relies on the willingness and ability of a bystander to effectively perform CPR and properly use a defibrillator. Time is of the essence when performing these life-saving measures.

PART TEN

Follow-up and Patient Care

CHAPTER 39

Patient Follow-up

Throughout this book I emphasize how important it is for you to establish an open and honest dialogue with your physician. Let your doctor know how you are feeling, and tell your doctor about any symptoms you may be experiencing. If it is your first visit to your heart doctor's office, he or she will complete a history, perform a physical examination, and do an ECG. Routine blood work and other diagnostic tests may be ordered, depending on your symptoms. Your physician will also review any current medications that you are taking, including over-the-counter drugs and supplements. Keep a current list of all your medications and the dosages you take in your wallet at all times. You might also carry a copy of a recent ECG wherever you go, because this document may help guide medical care should you develop cardiac symptoms.

Medical follow-up with your doctor is essential. If you have a heart condition or are at risk of a heart problem, getting good care and advice is absolutely necessary. A referral from a local and trusted doctor is often useful. Search the Web and see what information is available about doctors you are considering. Investigate their background, education, and professional experiences. Doing a good background check can help determine which one is a good choice for you. Once you meet the doctor, think about whether he or she satisfies your objectives regarding your health, respects your health care decisions, and has the time to answer your questions. Answering your questions is important, but if he or she is busy, don't be turned off. A busy doctor and practice may be a sign of the physician's success. You should also engage the nursing staff in conversation and get to know them, because nurses are often the first point of contact for patients.

Doctors follow up with patients with heart rhythm problems in several ways. If you are taking medications, you will need to see your physician routinely. As discussed in chapter 25, many drugs have side effects that can be serious, and many drugs can potentially interact adversely with other medications. Tell your doctor whether the medication is improving your symptoms or making them worse. Discuss with your doctor any supplements you add to your diet, such as fish oil, vitamins, garlic, red yeast rice, and herbal supplements.

Remote Monitoring of Implantable Devices

Patients with devices used to be seen personally in the doctor's office. Now, however, advances in technology make it possible for patients to submit their information remotely, by means of a telephone line, cable, satellite, or the Internet (see chapter 30). If you have a device, it may be possible to follow up through a remote monitoring service available through the device manufacturer. Web-based systems that provide home-based remote monitoring include Biotronik's Home Monitoring, Boston Scientific's Latitude, Medtronic's CareLink, and St. Jude Medical's Merlin.

To take advantage of the flexibility of this system, you must know how to set up your monitor and how to send a transmission. If you are going to send an unscheduled transmission, let your doctor and his or her staff know about your intention to do so. A remote transmission that occurs without the knowledge of the health care team is a prescription for a problem, since the strip you transmit may not be reviewed immediately. Remember, the remote transmission service is not a substitute for calling 911. If you are experiencing potentially life-threatening symptoms, call 911. *Do not* send an unscheduled transmission of data.

The process of sending the data from your device either directly or indirectly to your doctor's office is generally a regularly scheduled event. The doctor and the staff are expecting to receive the data. The monitoring system may include a wand that is placed over your device. Alternatively, this process may be performed by a form of wireless communication to a monitoring system (or base station) in your house or worn portably, using cellular technology. In any case, the data are obtained from the device and transmitted to a central station.

Alarms and alerts that are programmed by your doctor may trigger an alert on the monitoring Web site. The monitor and transmitter allow the device to communicate with a qualified health care provider in the physician's office, but not necessarily in real time. Most offices review their remote monitoring system only once a day, typically in the morning during office hours. A very serious alert received after hours might trigger a page to a member of the health care team, alerting them to an emergency device situation. The monitor is also useful in tracking when the battery on your device is running low.

Not every remote monitoring program is set up in the same way, so please check with your health care provider regarding their method of remote monitoring and their expectations regarding this service. In addition, your doctor may ask you to sign a paper that tells you what the service does and does not provide. Read carefully any documents you are asked to sign so that you fully understand the service and system that will be used. It is recommended that you call after making a transmission to verify that the correct party received the information. Usually a printout is generated in the physician's office, which is then reviewed by the physician. If you feel any seemingly non-life-threatening symptoms, *call the doctor's office.* He or she will determine whether more frequent transmissions are indicated, or whether you need to be seen in person.

How often do you need to see the doctor if you are being monitored remotely?

I believe that a patient should be seen at least once or twice yearly by the heart rhythm specialist (electrophysiologist) in the specialist's office. Without this kind of contact, it is easy for the patient to lose touch with the doctor and forget that the doctor has any oversight on their care. Do not hesitate to call your health care provider's office or make an appointment if you have any questions or concerns that you would like to address. If you are about to change physicians, call your current doctor's office to let them know. The office staff at the new doctor's office can help you set up your remote monitoring system for their office.

What should you tell your doctor?

Patients should never feel that their doctor does not have the time to listen to their concerns. If you feel this way consistently (rather than only occasionally, on a doctor's busy day), you may want to consider switching to a different doctor. Carry a list of current medications in your wallet at all times, including the name of each drug, the frequency and route of administration, and dosage. If you are unsure why you are taking a medication, ask your physician. Tell him or her about any change in medications, change in medical condition, or change in address. Most importantly, tell your doctor how you are feeling.

Call your physician's office if you have received a shock or shocking sensations related to the device. If you get more than two shocks from a defibrillator, call 911 for transport and go to the emergency room as soon as possible. Remember to carry your device identification card at all times.

If you have any side effects from any medication, do not hesitate to call your doctor. If you have any recurrence of symptoms following a heart rhythm procedure or if you develop side effects from medications or think that you are experiencing a complication, notify your doctor immediately and arrange follow-up.

CHAPTER 40

Support Groups

....

Information and support are available for patients and their families through organizations such as the Sudden Cardiac Arrest Association (www.suddencardiacarrest.org) and the Heart Rhythm Society (www.hrsonline.org). Support groups are beneficial for both individuals with heart disease and family members. The support groups provide education to keep patients and families up to date on current therapies, and they make it possible for individuals to express how they feel about their disease. In addition, they give families an opportunity to explore and understand the impact of the disease process on loved ones. For more information about some heart rhythm–related support groups, see table 40.1.

The American Heart Association (AHA) makes a number of publications available to patients and their families to help with their care and the management of their health. AHA family resources include help with diet and weight management and CPR classes in the community. The AHA can be easily accessed via the Web at www.heart.org.

Device companies have vast resources online. These resources include information regarding heart disease and arrhythmias, medications, catheter ablation, and devices. Access the manufacturers' Web sites at Biotronik (www.biotronik.com), Boston Scientific (www .bostonscientific.com), Medtronic (www.medtronic.com), and St. Jude Medical (www.sjm.com). Technical support telephone numbers for each of these device manufacturers are listed in table 40.2.

TABLE 40.1   *Heart rhythm–related support groups*

American Heart Association (www.heart.org): Helps support and advance the diagnosis and treatment of cardiovascular disease and stroke

Cardiac Arrhythmias Research and Education Foundation (www.longqt .org): Helps advocate for research and education in preventing sudden cardiac death

Heart Rhythm Society (www.hrsonline.org): A large international society for heart rhythm specialists (electrophysiologists) and ancillary and associated professionals as well as related personnel that supports all aspects of heart rhythm disorder understanding and advancement, including education, research, training, certification, treatment, and patient care and support

Hypertrophic Cardiomyopathy Association (www.4hcm.org): Helps support patients with hypertrophic cardiomyopathy and their families

Sudden Cardiac Arrest Association (www.suddencardiacarrest.org): Supports patients (and their families and friends) who have experienced or may be at risk for sudden cardiac arrest, with a focus on education in the prevention, resuscitation, and treatment of those at risk for sudden cardiac arrest

Sudden Arrhythmia Death Syndromes Foundation (www.sads.org): Offers support for inherited heart rhythm conditions such as long QT syndrome

TABLE 40.2   *Contact numbers for common device manufacturers*

Biotronik: 1-800-547-0394	Medtronic: 1-800-MEDTRON
Boston Scientific: 1-800-CARDIAC	St. Jude Medical: 1-800-PACEICD

CHAPTER 41

Defensive Patienting 101
A Primer on Patient Safety

··

Patient safety is the foremost concern of health care providers when they diagnose and treat heart rhythm patients. When receiving their degree from medical school, doctors take the Hippocratic oath, by which, among other provisions, they vow to do no harm. Even so, doctors and other health care workers are human, and unfortunately, humans make mistakes. Hospitals and medical clinics have protocols (checks and balances) to help ensure a patient's privacy and safety. But patients also need to have a system in place, much like defensive driving. This is what is sometimes called *defensive patienting*. Defensive patienting adds protection for you and helps you ensure your own safety. The following safety tips may help you in any number of health care situations.

First, competent adults who have unimpaired memories should be familiar with their own important medical information, and they should carry some of this information wherever they go (see table 41.1). The information kit begins with your full name and date of birth, to provide double identification. Ideally, the portable information will include a list of key medical conditions, all implanted devices and materials, allergies, and medications. You should also carry a copy of your most recent ECG. In addition, carry contact information, including the name of your health care proxy (the person who will make medical decisions for you if you become incapacitated). Should something unexpected happen to you, this portable medical information kit will provide any health care provider

TABLE 41.1 *Portable medical information kit*

1. Full name and date of birth
2. Medical conditions
3. Implantable devices and materials
4. Allergies
5. Medications
6. A copy of a recent ECG
7. Contact information, including a health care proxy

who comes to your aid with the basic essential medical information needed to expedite treatment. It is conceivable that eventually an electronic medical record system will be in place that makes carrying an information kit an unnecessary precaution. But at least for the short term, this list serves the same purpose as a portable electronic medical record system.

A second safety tip is to research hospitals, medical clinics, and doctors (see table 41.2). You can get information from doctors and from your friends and family members who have been treated by those institutions or individuals. In addition, you can search the Internet and employ a service such as HealthGrades (www.health grades.com), which supplies ratings of medical institutions and doctors along with other information about them. Organizations such as the Heart Rhythm Society (www.hrsonline.org) and the American Board of Internal Medicine (www.abim.org) provide useful information regarding board-certification status of heart rhythm specialists and other physicians.

A third safety tip is to do what's necessary to prepare for a test or procedure. For a summary of how you can protect your rights

TABLE 41.2 *Research the hospital and the doctor*

- Look into the experience of doctors and the experiences of other patients.
- Make use of services such as HealthGrades (www.healthgrades.com).
- Review information from the Heart Rhythm Society (www.hrsonline .org).
- Consult the American Board of Internal Medicine (www.abim.org).

and help avoid medical errors, see table 41.3. You must be aware of what is going on. You should make sure you are getting the right procedure on the correct part of the body by confirming this information with each new health care provider who approaches you. You need to be on your toes. Make sure you know and understand your condition and any tests that are ordered. What is involved in the tests? What are the risks, benefits, and alternatives? Did the doctor take time to explain these to you, and do you have any questions? If you do not understand something, it is your responsibility to stop and ask the questions. Question, question, question! And keep asking until your questions are answered to your satisfaction. Except in an emergency, do not go forward with any tests or procedures until you are satisfied that you understand the what, why, how, and by whom.

Tip number four: patients are entitled to privacy based on the Health Insurance Portability and Accountability Act (HIPAA). Doctors cannot disclose a patient's medical information to anyone, including family members and friends, without a patient's permission. A patient's medical information, including the medical record, is

TABLE 41.3 *Preparing for a test or procedure*

1. Be aware.
2. Know and understand what tests have been ordered.
3. Do not just go with the flow.
4. Prevent wrong patient, wrong procedure, wrong site procedures by actively participating in the safety processes:
    Double identification: This consists of staff checking your first name and last name plus your date of birth. Make sure they get the spelling and the dates right!
    Time out: Prior to any invasive procedure, a time out is required to confirm that the right patient, the right procedure, and the right site will be operated on (or will undergo a test or procedure). This must be performed with the entire medical team before proceeding.
5. Understand the risks, benefits, and alternatives before consenting to any test, procedure, or surgery.
6. *Question, question, question.*

private, and rules exist regarding with whom this information can be shared. For more information about HIPAA privacy rules, see www.hhs.gov/ocr/privacy/hipaa/understanding/index.html.

Finally, a patient who is not competent requires the input of a health care proxy to help make medical decisions. Ideally, a health care proxy is appointed by the patient in a legal document prepared *before* the patient is incompetent or has any need for the proxy. The proxy and all paperwork confirming that person's role as proxy need to be readily available and accessible. The proxy's contact information should be in the patient's medical chart. The contact information of important family members should also be readily available.

"Defensive Patienting 101" is a primer for protecting the patient in the complex medical network. Heart rhythm problems and procedures are intrinsically complicated. This book is intended to empower all patients and their family and friends to get the best care from their health care providers.

I hope this book will increase your understanding of your heart rhythm conditions and what you can do to optimize your treatment.

Acknowledgments

I thank all the Winthrop University Hospital staff members, summer students, and volunteers who reviewed and made editing suggestions in this book. I also thank Wendy Maltempi, Gerard Doorty, Alexandru Mitrache, Shanda Harris, Patricia Nadraus, Wilbur Asheld, and Ilyssa Scheinbach for their assistance. I would like to thank Brittany Cohen for her draft drawings, which demonstrated the heart's function and various heart rhythm abnormalities. I am also grateful to those who contributed their personal heart rhythm experiences to this book. In addition, I would like to thank Winthrop's CEO, John Collins, for his support of all my writing endeavors.

I greatly appreciate the endorsement of this book by the Sudden Cardiac Arrest Association. This charitable organization's mission is to advocate for patients and to help educate them about prevention, treatment, and resuscitation of sudden cardiac arrest. This education is certainly a major goal of this book.

Finally, I would like to thank Chris Chiames, executive director of the Sudden Cardiac Arrest Association, for his help in reviewing this manuscript as well as for his contribution of a foreword.

Appendix A

When an Electrophysiology Study Is Appropriate

....

1. To evaluate specific heart rhythm abnormalities (arrhythmias)
   a. slow heart rhythms (bradycardias)
   b. fast heart rhythms (tachycardias)
2. To evaluate heart rhythm treatments
   a. heart rhythm drugs (antiarrhythmic drugs)
   b. catheter ablation therapy
   c. heart rhythm (arrhythmia) surgery
   d. pacemaker function
   e. implantable cardioverter defibrillator (ICD) function
   f. other
3. To evaluate events or symptoms suggesting heart rhythm abnormalities (arrhythmias)
   a. cardiac arrest
   b. loss of consciousness (syncope)
   c. palpitations
4. To evaluate risk of rapid heart rhythms from the lower chambers of the heart (ventricular tachycardia or ventricular fibrillation)

Note: Be sure to talk with your doctor about any terms you do not completely understand.

Source: A. E. Buxton, H. Calkins, D. J. Callans, et al. "ACC/2006 Key Data Elements and Definitions for Electrophysiological Studies and Procedures." A report of the American College of Cardiology/Heart Association Task Force on Clinical Data Standards (ACC/Writing Committee to Develop Data Standards on Electrophysiology). *Journal of the American College of Cardiology* 48, no. 11 (2006): 2360–96.

Appendix B
When an Implantable Permanent Pacemaker Is Appropriate

....

1. Sinus node dysfunction with symptoms
2. Acquired high-grade atrioventricular block in an adult (Mobitz type II second-degree atrioventricular block or third-degree atrioventricular block/complete heart block)
3. Chronic bifascicular block with syncope and severe conduction disease at EP study
4. Nonreversible high-grade heart block following acute myocardial infarction
5. Hypersensitive carotid sinus syndrome and neurocardiogenic syncope
6. Cardiac transplantation
7. Neuromuscular disease
8. Sleep apnea syndrome with syncope and very long pauses on ECG
9. Cardiac sarcoidosis
10. Prevention and termination of atrial arrhythmias

Note: Be sure to talk with your doctor about any terms you do not completely understand.

Source: A. E. Epstein, J. P. DiMarco, K. A. Ellenbogen, et al. "ACC/AHA/HRS 2008 Guidelines for Device-Based Therapy of Cardiac Rhythm Abnormalities." A report of the American College of Cardiology/American Heart Association Task Force on Practice Guidelines (Writing Committee to Revise the ACC/AHA/NASPE 2002 Guideline Update for Implantation of Cardiac Pacemakers and Antiarrhythmia Devices) developed in collaboration with the American Association for Thoracic Surgery and Society of Thoracic Surgeons. *Journal of the American College of Cardiology* 51, no. 21 (2008): e1–62.

Appendix C

When an Implantable Cardioverter Defibrillator Is Appropriate

....

1. Secondary prevention (after an event)
    a. cardiac arrest and sustained ventricular tachycardia
    b. a short episode of ventricular tachycardia (nonsustained or less than 30 seconds) in a patient with an ischemic cardiomyopathy (coronary artery disease or heart attack and a weak heart muscle)
    c. cardiomyopathy of any type with symptoms of heart rhythm problems, including palpitations, light-headedness and dizziness, or loss of consciousness (syncope)
    d. syncope with inducible sustained ventricular tachycardia
2. Primary prevention (prior to an event, also called *prophylactic*)
    a. coronary artery disease
    b. non-ischemic dilated cardiomyopathy
    c. genetic syndromes such as long QT, short QT, Brugada syndromes
    d. hypertrophic cardiomyopathy
    e. right ventricular arrhythmogenic cardiomyopathy, or dysplasia
    f. noncompaction of the left ventricle
    g. catecholaminergic polymorphic ventricular tachycardia
    h. idiopathic ventricular tachycardia
    i. advanced heart failure and cardiac transplantation

Note: Be sure to talk with your doctor about any terms you do not completely understand.

Source: A. E. Epstein, J. P. DiMarco, K. A. Ellenbogen, et al. "ACC/AHA/HRS 2008 Guidelines for Device-Based Therapy of Cardiac Rhythm Abnormalities." A report of the American College of Cardiology/American Heart Association Task Force on Practice Guidelines (Writing Committee to Revise the ACC/AHA/NASPE 2002 Guideline Update for Implantation of Cardiac Pacemakers and Antiarrhythmia Devices) developed in collaboration with the American Association for Thoracic Surgery and Society of Thoracic Surgeons. *Journal of the American College of Cardiology* 51, no. 21 (2008): e1–62.

Appendix D
When Biventricular Therapy Is Appropriate

....

1. A combination of reasons, including each of the following:
   a. moderate to severe congestive heart failure (New York Heart Association class III or IV) despite treatment with optimal medical therapy (defined as at least a beta blocker and an angiotensin-converting enzyme inhibitor and/or an angiotensin II receptor blocker), unless the patient cannot tolerate these medications
   b. a left ventricular ejection fraction of 35 percent or less
   c. a wide QRS complex on ECG of more than 120 milliseconds
2. A combination including each of the following:
   a. asymptomatic or mild congestive heart failure (New York Heart Association class I or II) on optimal medical therapy
   b. a left ventricular ejection fraction of 30 percent or less
   c. a wide QRS complex on ECG of more than 130 milliseconds
3. Possibly after ablation of the AV junction in which the patient is paced 100 percent of the time (that is, the patient is pacemaker dependent)
4. According to a doctor's judgment, especially if the QRS is wide from pacing of the ventricle

Note: Be sure to talk with your doctor about any terms you do not completely understand.

Sources: 1. A. E. Epstein, J. P. DiMarco, K. A. Ellenbogen, et al. "ACC/AHA/HRS 2008 Guidelines for Device-Based Therapy of Cardiac Rhythm Abnormalities." A report of the American College of Cardiology/American Heart Association Task

Force on Practice Guidelines (Writing Committee to Revise the ACC/AHA/NASPE 2002 Guideline Update for Implantation of Cardiac Pacemakers and Antiarrhythmia Devices) developed in collaboration with the American Association for Thoracic Surgery and Society of Thoracic Surgeons. *Journal of the American College of Cardiology* 51, no. 21 (2008): e1–62.

2. Includes the results released from the MADIT-CRT (Multicenter Automatic Defibrillator Implantation Trial with Cardiac Resynchronization Therapy) study, which enrolled over 1,800 patients with either asymptomatic or mild heart failure (New York Heart Association class I and II), with an EF of 30 percent or less and a wide QRS complex. There was a 29 percent reduction in death or heart failure intervention when compared to standard ICDs in this study. A. J. Moss et al., "Cardiac-Resynchronization Therapy for the Prevention of Heart-Failure Events." *New England Journal of Medicine* 361, no. 14 (October 1, 2009): 1329–38.

Glossary

....

ablation: A procedure performed to get rid of, treat, and potentially cure a heart rhythm problem. See also **catheter ablation**

accessory pathway: An extra connection between the atrium and ventricle, in addition to the AV node.

acetylsalicylic acid (aspirin): An antiplatelet medication useful in preventing and treating a heart attack (myocardial infarction). Also part of a regimen used after stent placement.

alcohol septal ablation: A catheterization procedure in which alcohol is infused in a septal coronary artery branch to relieve the outflow tract obstruction seen in some forms of hypertrophic cardiomyopathy. See also **hypertrophic cardiomyopathy**

alpha blocker: A type of medication that blocks the alpha-adrenergic receptor. This medication may be used to treat high blood pressure, Raynaud disease, and benign prostatic hypertrophy (BPH). Medications may have both alpha- and beta-blocker properties and may be used to treat heart failure as well as high blood pressure.

amiodarone: A drug used to treat heart rhythm problems such as atrial fibrillation, atrial flutter, ventricular tachycardia, and ventricular fibrillation. Usually viewed as the strongest and most effective medication with the most side effects (can affect the eyes, skin, lungs, liver, and thyroid).

amyloidosis: A disease in which a protein called amyloid builds up in the heart and other organs. It can cause restrictive cardiomyopathy. See also **cardiomyopathy; restrictive cardiomyopathy**

angioplasty: A procedure in which a balloon catheter is placed into a coronary artery to open up a blocked blood vessel. See also **percutaneous coronary intervention**

angiotensin-converting enzyme inhibitor (ACE inhibitor): A medication used to treat high blood pressure and treat or prevent congestive heart failure.

angiotensin II receptor blocker (ARB): A medication used to treat high blood pressure and treat or prevent congestive heart failure.

antiarrhythmic drugs or medications: A type of drug or medication that may affect special channels within the cells (often sodium or potassium channels). These medications may be quite potent and often have the side effect of proarrhythmia in which a worse heart rhythm problem such as ventricular tachycardia may occur.

anticoagulant: Blood thinner used to prevent clot formation and stroke. This medication includes the oral version called warfarin (Coumadin) and the intravenous or subcutaneous injectable heparin (low-molecular-weight heparin).

arrhythmia: An abnormal heart rhythm.

arrhythmogenic right ventricular dysplasia (also called arrhythmogenic right ventricular cardiomyopathy, arrhythmogenic right ventricular cardiomyopathy/dysplasia, arrhythmogenic right ventricular dysplasia/cardiomyopathy, ARVD, ARVC, ARVC/D, or ARVD/C): A hereditary condition in which fat is deposited in the heart, typically in the right ventricle. Patients with this condition are predisposed to ventricular tachycardia.

asystole: A markedly slow heart rhythm (bradycardia) in which the heartbeat pauses for a prolonged period, usually much longer than 3 seconds.

atria: The upper chambers of the heart. There is a right and a left atrium.

atrial fibrillation: A very fast and irregular abnormal heart rhythm coming from the upper chambers of the heart (atria). Atrial fibrillation is often caused by triggers from within the pulmonary veins.

atrial flutter: An organized or regular fast heart rhythm coming from the upper chambers of the heart (atria).

automatic external defibrillator (AED): An external device, about the size of a lunch box, that is used to treat sudden cardiac arrest by shocking ventricular tachycardia or ventricular fibrillation. Patches are placed on the patient's chest, and the device provides audible prompts guiding the operator through a number of steps resulting in a shock (defibrillation) if necessary. These devices should be readily available in public places such as planes, stadiums, churches, temples, museums, and schools. See also **defibrillator; ventricular fibrillation; ventricular tachycardia**

AV node: A part of the heart's wiring system, which creates a delay for the electrical signal as it leaves the atria and conducts to the ventricles.

AV node reentry: A rapid rhythm involving an extra connection in the middle of the heart (the AV node).

beta blocker: A type of medication used to lower blood pressure, slow down a rapid heart rhythm, and prevent and treat heart failure and ischemia (the lack of blood flow to the heart). This medication blocks the beta-adrenergic receptor.

bifascicular block: A condition in which two of the three major fascicles of the heart's conduction system are blocked. These fasicles include the left anterior and posterior fascicles of the left bundle branch, and the right bundle branch, which is considered a single fascicle.

biventricular device: A device that paces (stimulates) both ventricles of the heart to improve its performance. This is also called cardiac resynchronization therapy (CRT) or biventricular pacing. See also **cardiac resynchronization therapy**

body mass index (BMI): This index can be used as an indicator of body fat. It is derived by one of the following formulas:

Using the metric system:
BMI (kg/m^2) = weight in kilograms ÷ (height in meters)^2
Using the English system:
BMI (kg/m^2) = weight in pounds × 703 ÷ (height in inches)^2

bradycardia: A slow heart rhythm, typically fewer than 60 beats per minute. Bradycardias may be significant when the heart rate is lower than 40 beats per minute, especially if the patient is symptomatic.

Brugada syndrome: A hereditary condition in which there are specific electrocardiographic findings and patients are at risk for sudden cardiac arrest.

bundle branch block: A condition diagnosed by an abnormal finding on the ECG, in which there is disease in at least one of the electrical branches that send electricity to the lower chambers of the heart. Typically, there is a right and a left bundle branch, and when a block or a delay occurs in either electrical structure, significant conduction disease may be present. An EP study may be useful in elucidating the amount of conduction disease.

calcium channel blockers: A type of medication that blocks the calcium channel and can cause a slow heart rate and a drop in blood pressure. It can be used to control rapid rhythms from the upper chambers (supraventricular tachycardia).

cardiac catheterization: A procedure in which a catheter (tube) is placed within the heart for diagnostic and/or therapeutic purposes. See also **coronary angiography; percutaneous coronary intervention; stent**

cardiac magnetic resonance imaging (MRI): A noninvasive procedure that may be used to visualize the heart and its surrounding structures.

cardiac output: The amount of blood pumped out of the heart in liters per minute. An indication of the strength of the heart along with the ejection fraction. See also **ejection fraction**

cardiac resynchronization therapy (CRT): The therapy provide by a biventricular pacing device. The timing of right and left ventricular pacing is performed to provide a more uniform (synchronous) ventricular contraction. See also **biventricular device**

cardiac tamponade: A compression that results when fluid builds up in the sac around the heart to the point that blood flow is impeded; the patient may have a potentially life-threatening drop in blood pressure, requiring abrupt removal of the fluid either by a needle or creation of a surgical pericardial window to relieve the tension. Cardiac tamponade may be the result of a perforation either from a needle, device wire or lead, or a heart catheter. In any case, emergency care is necessary to promptly treat this problem. See also **pericardial effusion**

cardiac transplantation (heart transplantation): A complicated surgical procedure in which a diseased heart is replaced by a healthy heart from a recently deceased patient.

cardiologist: A doctor who specializes in the heart.

cardiomyopathy: A weak heart muscle. This might be caused by various conditions, including but not limited to coronary artery disease (possibly including a heart attack), high blood pressure, valve disease, chemotherapy/radiation treatment, pregnancy, alcohol, hereditary conditions, infections, infiltrative conditions, and otherwise unknown causes.

cardiopulmonary resuscitation (CPR): A method of chest compressions and mouth-to-mouth ventilation to help resuscitate an unconscious patient in cardiac arrest.

cardioversion: A procedure performed to convert an abnormal heart rhythm back to a more normal rhythm. This can be performed with drugs (also called pharmacological cardioversion) or with electricity (electric shock, also called electrical cardioversion).

catheter ablation: A procedure in which a catheter is placed through a vein or artery to map, treat, and potentially cure a heart rhythm abnormality (arrhythmia). See also **ablation**

cholestyramine: A medication known as a bile acid sequestrant used to treat high cholesterol.

clofibrate: A medication from a group of medications known as fibrates that is used to treat high cholesterol and high triglycerides.

clopidogrel (Plavix): An antiplatelet medication used with acetylsalicylic acid (aspirin) following stent placement to prevent reocclusion of the coronary artery.

complete heart block (complete AV block or third-degree heart block): A condition in which the electrical activity from the upper chamber cannot conduct down to the lower chamber. All electrical activity from the upper chambers to the lower chambers is completely blocked.

computerized axial tomography (CT) angiogram: A test in which a patient is given contrast dye intravenously and then receives radiation to help doctors visualize the heart, its blood vessels, and surrounding structures. This test is also useful prior to an atrial fibrillation ablation procedure in visualizing the number and configuration of pulmonary veins that attach to the left atrium.

computer tomography angiography (CT angiography or CTA): A test in which contrast dye is administered to visualize the heart and its coronary arteries and determine whether blockages are present.

congestive heart failure (CHF or heart failure): A condition in which the heart fails to perform normally and fluid backs up into the lungs or other parts of the body. The patient may exhibit symptoms of fatigue, shortness of breath, leg swelling, and other forms of fluid accumulation.

coronary angiography (angiogram): A procedure in which a catheter is placed inside the heart and contrast dye administered to visualize the coronary arteries.

defensive patienting: The term used to describe how patients should protect their privacy and safety as they enter into medical care. It is analogous to defensive driving.

defibrillation: A procedure in which an electrical shock is delivered to the chest wall or internally to the heart to terminate an abnormally fast heart rhythm (tachycardia).

defibrillator: A device used to shock the patient's heart out of a very rapid rhythm (tachycardia) into a more normal rhythm.

digitalis: A medication that can help strengthen a weak heart in a patient with congestive heart failure. Can also be used to slow down heart rhythm problems such as rapidly conducting atrial fibrillation.

dilated cardiomyopathy: A weakening of the heart muscle in which part or all of the heart muscle dilates. See also **cardiomyopathy**

diuretic (water pill): A medication used to remove excess fluid that builds up in congestive heart failure. These drugs may alter electrolyte levels, such as potassium, and therefore blood needs to be periodically obtained to ensure that the electrolytes are within normal limits.

dofetilide: A heart rhythm drug that may be useful in treating atrial fibrillation and atrial flutter. This medication can worsen heart rhythm problems (such as by causing proarrhythmia). See also **proarrhythmia**

dronedarone: A heart rhythm drug that may be used to treat atrial fibrillation and atrial flutter. May be less effective than amiodarone, but also has less toxicity.

echocardiogram (echo): A test that uses sound waves (ultrasound) to visualize the heart, its structure, and its function. It is typically performed in two dimensions, showing cross-sections of the heart (called a two-dimensional echocardiogram). See also **transesophageal echocardiogram**

ejection fraction (EF): A measure of the function of the heart. EF can be determined by tests such as an echocardiogram, an angiogram, or a nuclear imaging study. In general, the ejection fraction is a measure of the fraction of blood ejected from the heart. An ejection fraction less than 50 percent is abnormal.

electrocardiogram (ECG or EKG): A test in which electrodes attached to the limbs and/or chest record electrical activity that is related to the heart, its rhythm, and its functionality.

electrophysiologist: A doctor who diagnoses and treats heart rhythm abnormalities. This doctor must train first in internal medicine and cardiology and subspecialize in the field of electrophysiology. An electrophysiologist may perform an EP study, a catheter ablation, or a device implant if warranted.

electrophysiology: The study of the electrical activity of the heart.

electrophysiology study (EP study): A procedure in which catheters are placed in veins (and occasionally in arteries) and threaded into the heart to study the electrical activity of the heart and to induce abnormal heart rhythms.

event recorder: A device used to record heart rhythm events in real time. Events are only recorded when the device is activated.

first-degree AV block: A form of heart block in which there is delay in the conduction from the atrium to the ventricle. A specific ECG pattern is observed.

flecainide: A heart rhythm medication useful in treating supraventricular tachycardias (including atrial fibrillation) in patients with structurally normal hearts.

gemfibrozil: A medication from a group known as fibrates that is used to treat high cholesterol and high triglycerides.

Health Insurance Portability and Accountability Act (HIPAA): Federal law that ensures the privacy of a patient's medical information.

heart transplantation: See **cardiac transplantation**

hemochromatosis: A disorder in which iron deposits in the body and its organs. It can cause a form of restrictive cardiomyopathy. See also **cardiomyopathy; restrictive cardiomyopathy**

high-grade AV block: A form of heart block in which electrical activity from the upper chambers is not consistently conducted to the lower chambers. In particular, more than one consecutive atrial beat fails to conduct to the lower chamber.

His bundle: Part of the wiring system of the heart that is below the AV node. If the His bundle is severely diseased, a patient may be at risk for heart block, and a pacemaker may be indicated.

HMG-CoA reductase inhibitors (statins): A class of medications useful in treating high cholesterol and to a lesser degree high triglycerides.

Holter monitor: A device used to record continuous heart rhythm information typically over one to two days.

hypertrophic cardiomyopathy: A condition in which the heart muscle is thickened and the heart's contraction may be very strong (hyperdynamic). A very thick heart muscle, significant family history of sudden death, the presence of ventricular tachycardia, or loss of consciousness (syncope) may all suggest the need for an implantable cardioverter defibrillator (ICD).

hypothyroidism: An endocrine or glandular condition in which the thyroid gland fails to produce enough thyroid hormone. As a result, the heart may beat very slowly, and occasionally, atrial fibrillation may occur. Treatment of a slow rhythm problem (bradycardia) may require medications such as thyroid hormone replacement.

ibutilide: An intravenous heart rhythm medication useful in treating atrial fibrillation and atrial flutter. May also cause proarrhythmia. See also **proarrhythmia**

implantable cardiac monitor (implantable loop recorder): An implantable device that can record heart rhythm–related information. Other physiological information might also be recorded.

implantable cardioverter defibrillator (ICD): A device that uses electrical energy to treat rapid and slow heart rhythms. High energy (DC energy) may be delivered to shock the patient out of a very fast rhythm (tachycardia).

informed consent: The process in which a doctor informs the patient of the risks, benefits, and alternatives to a given procedure. The patient should be given time to ask questions, and those questions should be answered to his or her satisfaction prior to consenting to a procedure.

INR (international normalized ration): A blood test used to determine how thin the blood is as a result of a patient being on warfarin (Coumadin).

interventionalist: A doctor who performs interventions (i.e., invasive procedures). With respect to the heart, an interventionalist typically performs cardiac catheterization, in which catheters are inserted into the heart and its arteries and contrast dye is delivered to visualize its structures. The doctor may decide to deliver a stent (piece of mesh metal) to keep a blockage open.

intracardiac echocardiography (ICE): A procedure in which a catheter is inserted into the heart to visualize internal structures, guide a transseptal procedure, and monitor for pericardial effusion formation (a possible complication from catheter ablation in which blood leaks into the sac around the heart).

ischemia: The lack of blood flow to the heart muscle itself.

ischemic cardiomyopathy: A weak heart muscle caused by the lack of blood flow to the heart (ischemia) or damage to the heart as the result of a heart attack (myocardial infarction).

lead extraction: A procedure to remove a pacemaker or defibrillator lead or leads from the heart. The procedure may involve special cutting tools that employ laser or radiofrequency energy.

left ventriculogram: A catheterization procedure in which a catheter is advanced into the left ventricle and contrast dye is injected to visualize the function of the left ventricle and calculate the ejection fraction. A similar procedure could be performed in the right ventricle, in which case it would be called a right ventriculogram. See also **ejection fraction**

long QT syndrome: A hereditary condition identified by abnormalities in the ECG and the patient's history, which may place the person at risk for ventricular tachycardia and sudden cardiac arrest.

loop recorder: A device used to record heart rhythm information. Once symptoms are identified and the device is activated, information that has been recorded is stored along with additional recorded data.

Lyme disease: A disease, following a tick bite, caused by a bacteria (*Borrelia burgdorferi*) found on a deer tick. This disease may result in slowing of the heart rate and heart block. In severe cases, myocarditis might also occur. Disease in the wiring system of the heart is usually restricted to the sinus and AV nodes and is typically reversible following treatment with antibiotics. See also **myocarditis**

magnetic resonance imaging (MRI): A test that uses strong magnetic fields to image the body, heart, and other organs.

mexiletine: A heart rhythm medication useful in treating ventricular tachycardia and ventricular fibrillation.

Mobitz type I second-degree heart block (Mobitz type I second-degree AV block or Wenckebach): A type of heart block that usually occurs in the AV node in which each atrial beat takes longer and longer to get to the ventricles until a beat is eventually blocked. If this rhythm is asymptomatic, it is not necessary to implant a pacemaker.

Mobitz type II second-degree heart block (Mobitz type II second-degree AV block): A type of heart block that may occur in the His bundle or below in which each atrial beat is followed by a ventricular beat in a regular sequence and then suddenly one atrial beat fails to conduct to the ventricle (a block occurs). The presence of this type of heart block often indicates the need for a permanent pacemaker.

myocardial infarction (heart attack): Irreversible damage to the heart muscle as the result of a blockage in an artery to the heart. May be an indicator for an implantable cardioverter defibrillator (ICD), especially if the ejection fraction is less than or equal to 30 percent.

myocarditis: An inflammation of the heart muscle, which may be caused by an infection (such as a bacteria or a virus) or an autoimmune condition (such as systemic lupus erythematosus). Myocarditis might also be found in some patients with peripartum cardiomyopathy. See also **peripartum dilated cardiomyopathy; systemic lupus erythematosus**

neurocardiogenic syncope: See **vasovagal syncope**

niacin (nicotinic acid): A medication used to treat high cholesterol and high triglycerides.

nonfluoroscopic three-dimensional mapping: A method used during an EP study to help identify the location of heart rhythm problems along with the position of catheters within the heart.

NPO (*nil per os*): Means "nothing by mouth." Typically patients must have nothing to eat or drink for at least 6 hours prior to any procedure. Medications with a sip of water may be permitted. Please ask your doctor for specific instructions.

NSAIDs: Nonsteroidal anti-inflammatory drugs such as ibuprofen, which may interfere with certain medications. Please talk to your doctor prior to taking this type of treatment along with your heart medications.

pacemaker: A device that is implanted to treat slow heart rhythms (bradycardias). It can also be used to treat heart failure. It is a component of an implantable cardioverter defibrillator (ICD).

percutaneous coronary intervention (PCI): A procedure that is performed to open up a blocked coronary artery. A balloon catheter is placed across the blocked vessel to open up the blockage. A stent (expandable piece of metal) may then be inserted to keep the coronary artery open. See also **angioplasty; stent**

pericardial effusion: The presence of blood or fluid in the pericardial sac around the heart. This may be the result of a cardiac perforation, in which blood may flow into the sac. If blood continues to flow into the pericardial sac, it may put pressure on the heart muscle itself and potentially prevent blood from leaving the heart. If the latter occurs, the patient may have a life-threatening condition called cardiac tamponade, which requires immediate treatment. See also **cardiac tamponade**

peripartum dilated cardiomyopathy: A cardiomyopathy of unknown etiology occurring around the time of pregnancy. Myocarditis may be seen in many patients with this disorder. See also **myocarditis**

presyncope: Light-headedness and dizziness short of true loss of consciousness. The feeling that one is going to "black out" without actually blacking out.

proarrhythmia: A side effect of a medication or device in which a rhythm problem is worsened or exacerbated. A drug such a procainamide may cause a form of ventricular tachycardia called *torsades de pointes*. Treatment is often to stop the trigger through other medications such as lidocaine; even pacing therapy may be necessary. See also *torsades de pointes*

procainamide: A heart rhythm medication used occasionally in intravenous form to provoke ECG changes seen in Brugada syndrome. Infrequently used as a treatment of heart rhythm problems due to the presence of more efficacious medications with fewer side effects (including proarrhythmia). See also **proarrhythmia**

propafenone: A medication used to treat atrial fibrillation and atrial flutter, especially in a patient with a structurally normal heart. Proarrhythmia may be a side effect. See also **proarrhythmia**

pulmonary vein isolation (PVI): A catheter ablation procedure in which the pulmonary veins are electrically isolated from the left atrium to prevent the trigger for atrial fibrillation (which is often within the pulmonary vein itself) from initiating atrial fibrillation.

Purkinje fibers: Specialized electrical tissue that helps to conduct electrical signals from the His bundle to the ventricular muscles.

QT dispersion: A measurement obtained from a standard ECG that can give useful information related to the risk for developing ventricular tachycardia.

Raynaud disease: A vascular disorder in which blood flow is impeded as a result of exposure to cold or stress. Fingers, toes, ear lobes, and the nose may turn pale as a result.

recall: The term used when a repetitive problem is identified with a device or one of its components. The specific action taken by the manufacturer, the United States Food and Drug Administration, and doctors will depend on how critical the problem is.

restrictive cardiomyopathy: A form of heart muscle weakness in which the ventricles are stiff and cannot fill properly. Often caused by the buildup of a protein called amyloid. See also **amyloidosis; cardiomyopathy**

septal myotomy-myomectomy: A surgical procedure in which a part of the heart muscle is surgically removed to relieve the obstruction that may be found in some forms of hypertrophic cardiomyopathy. See also **hypertrophic cardiomyopathy**

signal-averaged ECG (SAECG): A specialized ECG that can give useful information related to the risk for developing ventricular tachycardia.

sinus node (sinoatrial node, SA node): The start of the electricity in the heart, high up in the right atrium.

sotalol: A heart rhythm medication useful in treating atrial fibrillation, atrial flutter, ventricular tachycardia, and ventricular fibrillation. This medication can also cause or worsen life-threatening heart rhythm problems such as ventricular tachycardia and ventricular fibrillation (proarrhythmia). See also **proarrhythmia**

statins: See **HMG-CoA reductase inhibitors**

stent: A piece of mesh metal deployed inside a coronary artery across a blockage to keep the blockage open. The stent may be made of bare metal or coated with drugs (drug-eluting stents, or DES) to prevent restenosis. The placement of a stent may also be referred to as stenting. See also **angioplasty; percutaneous coronary intervention**

stress echocardiogram: A form of stress test in which wall-motion abnormalities may be visualized by echocardiogram (indicating a blocked artery or damaged heart muscle) following exercise or drug-induced stress to a patient. See also **echocardiogram**

stress test: A procedure in which the body is stressed either by exercise or medications to determine how well the heart is functioning. The test is often useful in determining the presence of blocked coronary arteries and whether a person has had a heart attack (myocardial infarction).

sudden cardiac arrest: The number one killer. Usually caused by a rapid heart rhythm from the lower chambers of the heart (ventricles), called ventricular tachycardia or ventricular fibrillation.

supraventricular: Above the ventricle.

supraventricular tachycardia (SVT): A rapid heart rhythm occurring above the ventricle (typically in the atria or AV node).

syncope: Loss of consciousness. See also **presyncope; tilt table test; vasovagal syncope**

systemic lupus erythematosus: An autoimmune disorder that affects the joints, skin, lungs, kidneys, nervous system, and heart. It may cause myocarditis. See also **myocarditis**

tachycardia: A rapid heart rhythm with rates of 100 beats per minute or more. At rest, tachycardias may be abnormal, depending on the circumstance, when the heart rate exceeds 120 beats per minute.

tilt table test: A simple procedure in which a patient is strapped to a table and then tilted almost upright (typically between 60 to 80 degrees) for up to 45 minutes to determine the cause of syncope or presyncope. Heart rate and blood pressure are monitored during the procedure, and in some cases a medication may be infused to facilitate the procedure. See also **presyncope; syncope; vasovagal syncope**

torsades de pointes: A serious form of ventricular tachycardia caused by medications that lengthen the QT interval or by the hereditary long QT syndrome. The ventricular tachycardia appears to be turning or twisting about an axis. See also **long QT syndrome**

transesophageal echocardiogram: A procedure in which a tube containing an echo probe is inserted down the esophagus to view specific structures in and around the heart. It is particularly useful in defining the presence of blood clots in the left atrial appendage (a spot not well seen by a standard echocardiogram). This procedure is frequently performed prior to cardioverting atrial fibrillation, especially if the patient has been in atrial fibrillation for some time and has not been well anticoagulated. See also **echocardiogram**

transseptal procedure: A procedure that uses a needle to puncture the tissue that separates the right and left atrium (atrial septum) to advance a catheter from the right side of the heart into the left side (left atrium or ventricle). This procedure is a standard part of a routine atrial fibrillation procedure such as pulmonary vein isolation.

T-wave alternans (TWA): A test to help determine a patient's risk for sudden death. This test is often performed with a special computer during a stress test.

universal protocol: The Joint Commission on Accreditation of Healthcare Organizations national patient safety goals in order to prevent wrong patient, wrong site, and wrong surgery procedures. The process includes a preprocedure verification, including double identification to determine the correct patient, marking of the procedural site by a licensed practitioner, and the performance of a "time out" immediately before initiating the procedure. The time out allows all parties to review that the patient, procedure, and procedural site are correct and that all important documents and equipment are in place prior to initiating the procedure.

vasovagal syncope (neurocardiogenic syncope): A common type of fainting, or syncope (loss of consciousness), often triggered by standing for a long period, in which the blood pressure (and possibly the heart rate) drops precipitously.

ventricular fibrillation (VF): A very rapid and irregular rhythm from the lower chamber or chambers of the heart (ventricles), which may cause sudden cardiac arrest. If this rhythm problem is not immediately terminated, sudden death may result.

ventricular tachycardia (VT): A rapid rhythm from the lower chamber or chambers of the heart (ventricles), which may cause sudden cardiac arrest.

warfarin (Coumadin): A medication used to prevent the formation of blood clots in the heart and to prevent stroke in patients with conditions such as atrial fibrillation and atrial flutter. Warfarin can also be used to treat clots in other blood vessels and in the lungs, and to prevent clotting in people with mechanical heart valves. This medication must be carefully monitored by a blood test called an INR. The major side effect is increased bleeding tendency. See also **INR**

Wolff-Parkinson-White (WPW) syndrome: A condition in which there is an extra connection between the upper and lower chambers of the heart (called an accessory pathway). Patients with this condition often have a specific ECG finding called a delta wave and are symptomatic with palpitations, light-headedness and dizziness, or loss of consciousness. This condition can be readily treated by catheter ablation.

Bibliography

"2005 American Heart Association Guidelines for Cardiopulmonary Resuscitation and Emergency Cardiovascular Care." *Circulation* 112, supplement 1 (2005): IV-1–211.

Augderheide, T., M. F. Hazinski, G. Nicho, et al. "Community Lay Rescuer Automated External Defibrillation Programs. Key State Legislative Components and Implementation Strategies. A Summary of a Decade of Experience for Healthcare Providers, Policymakers, Legislators, Employers, and Community Leaders from the American Heart Association Emergency Cardiovascular Care Committee, Council on Clinical Cardiology, and Office of State Advocacy." *Circulation* (2006) DOI: 10.1161/CIRCULATIONAHA.106.172289.

Blomström-Lundqvist, C., M. M. Scheinman, E. M. Aliot, et al. "ACC/Guidelines for the Management of Patients with Supraventricular Arrhythmias—Executive Summary." A report of the American College of Cardiology/American Heart Association Task Force on Practice Guidelines (Writing Committee to Develop Guidelines for the Management of Patients with Supraventricular Arrhythmias). *Circulation* 108 (2003):1871–1909.

Buxton, A. E., H. Calkins, D. J. Callans, et al. "ACC/2006 Key Data Elements and Definitions for Electrophysiological Studies and Procedures." A report of the American College of Cardiology/Heart Association Task Force on Clinical Data Standards (ACC/Writing Committee to Develop Data Standards on Electrophysiology). *Journal of the American College of Cardiology* 48, no. 11 (2006): 2360–96.

Calkins, H., J. Brugada, D. L. Packer, et al. "HRS/EHRA/ECAS Expert Consensus Statement on Catheter and Surgical Ablation of Atrial Fibrillation: Recommendations for Personnel, Policy, Procedures and Follow-up." A report of the Heart Rhythm Society (HRS) Task Force on Catheter and Surgical Ablation of Atrial Fibrillation. *Heart Rhythm* 4 (2007): 816–61.

Cohen, T. J. *Practical Electrophysiology.* 2nd ed. Malvern, PA: HMP Communications, 2009, 1–349.

Epstein, A. E., J. P. DiMarco, K. A. Ellenbogen, et al. "ACC/AHA /HRS 2008 Guidelines for Device-Based Therapy of Cardiac Rhythm Abnormalities." A report of the American College of Cardiology/American Heart Association Task Force on Practice Guidelines (Writing Committee to Revise the ACC/AHA/NASPE 2002 Guideline Update for Implantation of Cardiac Pacemakers and Antiarrhythmia Devices) developed in collaboration with the American Association for Thoracic Surgery and Society of Thoracic Surgeons. *Journal of the American College of Cardiology* 51, no. 21 (2008): e1–62.

Fuster, V., L. E. Ryden, D. S. Cannom, et al. "ACC/ESC 2006 Guidelines for the Management of Patients with Atrial Fibrillation." A report of the American College of Cardiology/American Heart Association Task Force on Practice Guidelines and the European Society of Cardiology Committee for Practice Guidelines (Writing Committee to Revise the 2001 Guidelines for the Management of Patients with Atrial Fibrillation), developed in collaboration with the European Heart Rhythm Association and the Heart Rhythm Society. *Circulation* 114 (2006): e257–e354.

Goldberger, J. J., M. E. Cain, S. H. Hohnloser, et al. "American Heart Association/American College of Cardiology Foundation/Heart Rhythm Society Scientific Statement on Noninvasive Risk Stratification Techniques for Identifying Patients at Risk for Sudden Cardiac Death." A scientific statement from the American Heart Association Council on Clinical Cardiology Committee on Electrocardiography and Arrhythmias and Council on Epidemiology and Prevention. *Circulation* 118 (2008): 1497–1518.

Hendel, R. C., D. S. Berman, M. F. Di Carli, et al., "ACCF/ASNC/ACR /AHA/ASE/SCCT/SCMR/SNM 2009 Appropriate Use Criteria for Radionuclide Imaging." A report of the American College of Cardiology Foundation Appropriate Use Criteria Task Force, the American Society of Nuclear Cardiology, the American College of Radiology, the American Heart Association, the American Society of Echocardiography, the Society of Cardiovascular Computed Tomography, the Society for Cardiovascular Magnetic Resonance, and the Society of Nuclear Medicine. Endorsed by the American College of Emergency Physicians. *Circulation* 119 (2009): e561–e587.

Hohnloser, S. H., H. J. G. M. Crijns, M. van Eickels, et al. "Effect of Dronedarone on Cardiovascular Events in Atrial Fibrillation." *New England Journal of Medicine* 360 (2009): 668–78.

Jessup, M., W. T. Abraham, D. E. Casey, et al. "2009 Focused Update: ACCF/AHA Guidelines for the Diagnosis and Management of Heart Failure in Adults." A report of the American College of Cardiology Foundation/American Heart Association Task Force on Practice Guidelines, developed in collaboration with the International Society for Heart and Lung Transplantation. *Circulation* 119 (2009): 1977–2016.

Kadish, A. H., A. E. Buxton, H. L. Kennedy, et al. "ACC/AHA Clinical Competence Statement on Electrocardiography and Ambulatory Electrocardiography." A report of the ACC/AHA/ACP–ASIM Task Force on Clinical Competence (ACC/AHA Committee to Develop a Clinical Competence Statement on Electrocardiography and Ambulatory Electrocardiography). Endorsed by the International Society for Holter and Noninvasive Electrocardiology. *Circulation* 104 (2001): 3169–78.

Moss, A. J., et al. "Cardiac-Resynchronization Therapy for the Prevention of Heart-Failure Events." *New England Journal of Medicine* 361, no. 14 (October 1, 2009): 1329–38.

Strickberger, S. A., D. W. Benson, I. Biaggioni, et al. "AHA/Scientific Statement on the Evaluation of Syncope." From the American Heart Association Councils on Clinical Cardiology, Cardiovascular Nursing, Cardiovascular Disease in the Young, and Stroke, and the Quality of Care and Outcomes Research Interdisciplinary Working Group; and the American College of Cardiology Foundation, in collaboration with the Heart Rhythm Society. Endorsed by the American Autonomic Society. *Circulation* 113 (2006): 316.

Strickberger, S. A., J. Conti, E. G. Daoud, et al. "AHA Science Advisory. Patient Selection for Cardiac Resynchronization Therapy." From the Council on Clinical Cardiology Subcommittee on Electrocardiography and Arrhythmias and the Quality of Care and Outcomes Research Interdisciplinary Working Group, in collaboration with the Heart Rhythm Society. *Circulation* 11 (2005): 2146–50.

Tracy, C. M., M. Akhtar, J. P. DiMarco, et al. "American College of Cardiology/American Heart Association 2006 Update of the Clinical Competence Statement on Invasive Electrophysiology Studies, Catheter Ablation, and Cardioversion." A report of the American College of Cardiology/American Heart Association/American College of Physicians Task Force on Clinical Competence and Training, developed in collaboration with the Heart Rhythm Society. *Circulation* 114 (2006): 1654–68.

Wilkoff, B. L., C. J. Love, C. L. Byrd, et al. "Transvenous Lead Extraction: Heart Rhythm Society Expert Consensus on Facilities, Training, Indications, and Patient Management." Developed in collaboration with the American College of Cardiology and the American Heart Association. *HeartRhythm* (July 2009): 1085–1104.

Zipes, D. P., A. J. Camm, M. Borggrefe, et al. "ACC/2006 Guidelines for Management of Patients with Ventricular Arrhythmias and the Prevention of Sudden Cardiac Death." A report of the American College of Cardiology/American Heart Association Task Force and the European Society of Cardiology Committee for Practice Guidelines (Writing Committee to Develop Guidelines for Management of Patients with Ventricular Arrhythmias and the Prevention of Sudden Cardiac Death), developed in collaboration with the European Heart Rhythm Association and the Heart Rhythm Society. *Circulation* 114 (2006): e385–484.

Index

anticoagulants, 94, 96, 98, 184; for
ablation procedures, 87; for atrial
fibrillation / atrial flutter, 31, 34,
36, 38, 99–100; stopping before
stress test, 64
antihypertensive drugs, 98
antiplatelet medications: and atrial
fibrillation, 31, 99–100; for coronary artery disease, 97; and stents,
99; stopping before stress test,
64–65
antitachycardia pacing, 109
aorta, 4–7
aortic stenosis, 54
aortic valve, 4, 6, 137
ARBs. *See* angiotensin II receptor
blockers
arrhythmias, 13–14, 184; automatic
external defibrillator for, 46,
160–62; bradycardias, 21–23, 43;
cardiac arrest due to, 43–44; and
cardiomyopathy, 135; catheter ablation for, 87–89; death from, 27;
during electrophysiology study, 81;
and genetic disorders, 142; and hypertrophic cardiomyopathy, 140;
medications for, 94–96; monitoring for, 66–67, 117–18; symptoms
of, 14; ventricular, 27–29
arrhythmogenic right ventricular dysplasia, 71–72, 138, 139, 143, 184
arteries, 10; coronary, 7
ARVD. *See* arrhythmogenic right
ventricular dysplasia
aspirin, 31. *See also* acetylsalicylic
acid
asystole, 22, 23, 44, 184
atherosclerosis, 44–45, 99, 136
atria, 3–6, 184
atrial fibrillation, 14, 24, 26, 31, 32–
37, 184; biventricular pacing for,
116; catheter ablation for, 34–36,
89; and electrocardiogram, 61;
facts about, 35; medications for,
31, 32, 34, 94–96, 99–100; paroxysmal, 35; risk factors for, 32–33;

stroke and, 31, 32, 34, 99; and
transesophageal echocardiogram,
68, 195; treatment of, 34–36
atrial flutter, 24, 26, 31, 37–39, 184;
electrocardiogram in, 38, 61; facts
about, 39; medications for, 37–38,
95, 99–100; treatment of, 37–38
atrial tachycardia, 24–25, 31
atrioventricular node, 3, 5, 13, 185
automatic external defibrillators, 46,
148, 160–62, 184–85; locations of,
46, 160; users of, 160–62; work-
ings of, 161
AV junction ablation, 36
AV node. *See* atrioventricular node
AV node reentrant tachycardia, 30
AV node reentry, 185

beta blockers, 93, 94–96, 185; and
atrial fibrillation, 100; and biventricular devices, 116; bradycardia
induced by, 21; for coronary artery disease, 97, 99; and dilated
cardiomyopathy, 139; for heart
failure, 97, 100–101, 133, 181; for
hypertension, 98; and hypertrophic
cardiomyopathy, 140; and long
QT syndrome, 144, 147, 148; and
restrictive cardiomyopathy, 141
bifascicular block, 178, 185
Biotronik: Home Monitoring system,
166; telephone number for, 170;
Web site for, 169
biventricular devices, 114–16, 185;
after AV node ablation, 116; benefits of, 115, 116, 134; complications with, 116, 122-124; eligibil-
ity for, 114–15, 134; indications
for, 181; and medications, 116
blood flow, 5–7, 10
blood pressure, high, 32, 33, 46, 47,
153; medications for, 93, 94-95,
97, 98. *See also* hypertension
blood thinners. *See* anticoagulants
BMI. *See* body mass index
body mass index, 153, 154, 185

Boston Scientific: Latitude system, 166; telephone number for, 170; Web site for, 169

bradycardia, 14, 21–23, 59, 185; cardiac arrest due to, 43–44; causes of, 21–22; medication-induced, 21; occult, 118; pacemaker for, 23, 44, 105; sinus, 22–23, 61; symptoms of, 21, 23; during tilt table test, 82; types of, 23

Brugada syndrome, 143, 145–46, 179, 185

bundle branch block, 114, 185–86

caffeine, 147

calcium channel blockers, 95, 96, 186; and atrial fibrillation, 100; bradycardia induced by, 21; for hypertension, 98; for hypertrophic cardiomyopathy, 140; for restrictive cardiomyopathy, 141

cardiac amyloidosis, 141

cardiac arrest. *See* sudden cardiac arrest

Cardiac Arrhythmias Research and Education Foundation, 170

cardiac catheterization, 64, 73–76, 186; case example of, 75–76; recovery after, 75; risks of, 75

cardiac cycle, 13

cardiac imaging, 8, 71–72; coronary angiogram, 15, 44, 64, 73–74, 112, 188; CT angiogram, 8, 71, 72, 187; and dye allergy, 71, 73; echocardiogram, 68–70; MRI, 8, 15, 71–72, 186

cardiac life support, 12

cardiac monitors, 8, 54, 66–67; implantable, 66–67, 117–18

cardiac output, 15, 186

cardiac rehabilitation, 9

cardiac resynchronization therapy, 114, 181, 186. *See also* biventricular devices

cardiac tamponade, 186, 193

cardiac transplantation, 186

cardiac ultrasound. *See* echocardiogram

cardiologists, 8–9, 57, 186; asking questions of, 173; choosing a doctor, 165–66; information to share with, 168; patient relationship with, 165; researching, 172; subspecialties of, 8–9; training of, 8

cardiomyopathy, 135–41, 186–87; dilated, 135, 136–39, 188; hypertrophic, 16, 17, 135, 139–40, 143, 144, 190; ICD for, 179; restrictive, 135, 141, 194; symptoms of, 135

cardiopulmonary resuscitation, 12, 46–47, 148, 155–59, 187; ABCs of, 155–56; assessing need for, 156–57; learning, 46, 160–62; performing, 156–59; training in, 47, 155–56

cardiothoracic surgeon, 9

cardioversion, 81, 90–92, 187; chemical, 92; compared with defibrillation, 90; electrical, 90; indications for, 91; paddle placement for, 90, 91

CareLink (Medtronic), 166

carotid pulse, 10, 157

carvedilol, 97

catheter ablation, 4, 87–89, 187; of accessory pathway, 25, 30; and atrial fibrillation, 34–36, 89; and atrial flutter, 31, 37; and AV node reentrant tachycardia, 30; biventricular pacing after, 116; conditions treated by, 87, 88; echocardiogram during, 69–70; during electrophysiology study, 78–79, 87; equipment for, 87, 88; and hereditary conditions, 147; procedure for, 87–88; risks of, 87; success rates for, 88–89; and supraventricular tachycardia, 89; and ventricular tachycardia, 89

catheters, 8, 9

CHADS2, 34

chemotherapy-induced cardiomyopathy, 137, 139

ders, 146–47; left ventriculogram, 74, 191; percutaneous coronary, 74–76; preparation for, 172–73; stress, 63–65; tilt table, 53, 54, 82–83, 195; T-wave alternans, 77, 195

diet, 46, 112, 141, 153

dietary supplements, 166

digitalis, 188; bradycardia induced by, 21; for heart failure, 98, 101, 134

dilated cardiomyopathy, 135, 136–39, 188; alcohol-related, 137–38; and arrhythmogenic right ventricular dysplasia, 138; cancer treatment–related, 137; causes of, 136–38; heart failure due to, 136; hypertensive, 137; idiopathic, 137; from inflammation or infection, 138; ischemic, 136–37, 191; peripartum, 137, 193; treatment of, 138–39; valvular, 137

diuretics, 188; and biventricular devices, 116; for heart failure, 98, 101, 134; and long QT syndrome, 144; and restrictive cardiomyopathy, 141

dizziness, 14, 21, 23, 26, 32, 54, 82, 105, 117, 133, 135

DNA, 142

dobutamine, 64

doctor-patient relationship, 165

dofetilide, 95, 96, 100, 188

driving, 121, 122

dronedarone, 95, 96, 100, 188

dye allergy, 71, 73

ECG. *See* electrocardiogram

echocardiogram, 8, 15, 68–70, 188; during catheter ablation, 69–70; facts about, 69; stress and, 64, 69, 194; transesophageal, 68, 195

EF. *See* ejection fraction

ejection fraction, 15–17, 188; calculation of, 15–16; and devices, 114; facts about, 16; with hypertrophic

cardiomyopathy, 16, 17; ICD and, 16–17, 47; low, 16, 17, 47, 110; normal, 16

EKG. *See* electrocardiogram

electrical impulses, 3–4, 13

electrocardiogram, 59–62, 188–89; and atrial fibrillation, 61; and atrial flutter, 38, 61; and Brugada syndrome, 146; carrying copy of, 165, 171; facts about, 59; and hereditary disorders, 146; and long QT syndrome, 144, 148; of normal sinus rhythm, 25, 59, 60; signal-averaged, 146, 194; and sinus bradycardia, 22–23, 61; during stress test, 63; and supraventricular tachycardia, 26; and ventricular tachycardia, 62; waveforms on, 60–61; and Wolff-Parkinson-White syndrome, 62

electrophysiologists, 8, 57, 78, 189

electrophysiology, 189

electrophysiology study, 8, 78–81, 113, 189; catheter ablation and, 78–79, 87; indications for, 79–80, 177; lab for, 78, 79; nonfluoroscopic 3-D mapping during, 192; procedure for, 79; risks of, 80; terminating arrhythmias during, 81

EP study. *See* electrophysiology study

errors, medical, 173

event recorder, 66, 67, 189

exercise, 9, 153; decreased tolerance for, 132–33; heart rate during, 24; and long QT syndrome, 144, 148

fainting. *See* syncope

family history of heart disease, 153–54; case example of, 147–49

fascicles, 185

fatigue, 15, 21, 23, 32, 133

femoral pulse, 10

first-degree AV block, 189

flecainide, 95, 96, 100, 189

fluid pills. *See* diuretics

fluoroscopy, 78

follow-up, 165–68; for medication monitoring, 166; after pacemaker implantation, 108; remote monitoring of implantable devices, 121–22, 166–68

gemfibrozil, 97, 99, 189
gene therapy, 147
genetic disorders. *See* hereditary cardiac disorders
Genetic Information Nondiscrimination Act, 146
genetic testing, 146–47, 148
grapefruit and grapefruit juice, 93

HCM. *See* hypertrophic cardiomyopathy
health care proxy, 174
HealthGrades, 172
Health Insurance Portability and Accountability Act, 173–74, 189
heart: blood flow through, 5–7; contraction of, 10; facts about, 7; infections of, 138; pumping action of, 15, 114, 135; structure of, 3, 4
heart attack. *See* myocardial infarction
heart block, 13, 22–23, 59–60; first-degree AV, 189; high-grade AV, 189; pacemaker for, 23; second-degree, 22, 23, 178, 191–92; third-degree (complete), 22, 23, 187
heart failure, 9, 131–34; and biventricular devices, 114–16, 134, 181; causes of, 133; classes of, 132; diagnostic tests for, 133; diastolic, 131, 132; from dilated cardiomyopathy, 136; ICD for, 110; impaired blood pumping in, 114, 131; implantable cardioverter defibrillator for, 134; left, 131; management of, 133–34; medications for, 97–98, 100–101, 133–34; and remodeling, 131; right, 131; symptoms of, 15, 132–33; systolic, 131, 132
heart failure specialists, 9

heart muscle disease. *See* cardiomyopathy
heart rate, 7, 10–11; during exercise, 24
heart rhythm, 13; abnormal, 13–14 (*see also* arrhythmias); fast, 4, 11–14, 24–26, 59 (*see also* tachycardia); irregular, 14; normal, 11, 12, 13, 24, 25, 59, 60; slow, 4, 14, 21–23, 59 (*see also* bradycardia)
Heart Rhythm Society, 79, 94, 105, 119, 144, 169, 170, 172
hemochromatosis, 141, 189
heparin, 184. *See also* anticoagulants
hereditary cardiac disorders: arrhythmogenic right ventricular dysplasia, 71–72, 138, 139, 143; Brugada syndrome, 143, 145–46; case example of, 147–49; diagnostic tests for, 142–49, 146–47; hypertrophic cardiomyopathy, 16, 17, 135, 139–40, 143, 144; long QT syndrome, 143–45; treatment of, 147
high-grade AV block, 189
HIPAA. *See* Health Insurance Portability and Accountability Act
Hippocratic Oath, 171
His bundle, 3, 5, 13, 189
His-Purkinje system, 3–4, 13
HMG-CoA reductase inhibitors, 99, 189, 194; for atrial fibrillation, 32, 34; and coronary artery disease, 97; and dilated cardiomyopathy, 138
holiday heart, 138
Holter monitor, 66, 67, 190
Home Monitoring (Biotronik), 166
hospitals, 172
hydralazine, 101
hypertension, 31, 33, 34, 35, 93, 98, 137, 153; medications for, 93, 96. *See also* blood pressure, high
hypertensive cardiomyopathy, 137, 139
hypertrophic cardiomyopathy, 135,

malfunction of implantable devices, 124, 126–27; isolated component failure, 126; recalls due to, 120, 127, 193–94; safety advisory about, 120, 127
maze procedure, 36
medical information kit, 171–72
medications, 93–101; allergies to, 94; antiarrhythmic drugs, 94–96; for atrial fibrillation / atrial flutter, 31, 32, 34, 37–38, 99–100; and biventricular devices, 116; carrying list of, 101, 165, 168; for coronary artery disease, 96–97, 99; and dilated cardiomyopathy, 139; drug or food interactions with, 93, 94; for heart failure, 97–98, 100–101, 133–34, 181; and hereditary conditions, 147; for high blood pressure, 93, 94-95, 97, 98; for high cholesterol, 32, 97, 99, 153, 154, 187, 189, 192; how to take, 93–94; for hypertension, 93, 96, 98; for hypertrophic cardio-myopathy, 140; and long QT syndrome, 144–45, 147, 148; monitoring of, 166; principles for use of, 93–94; for restrictive cardiomyopathy, 141; side effects of, 94, 166, 168; before stress tests, 64–65; types of, 95, 97–98; for ventricular arrhythmias, 100
Medtronic: CareLink system, 166; telephone number for, 170; Web site for, 169
Merlin (St. Jude Medical), 166
mexiletine, 95, 96, 100, 191
mini-stroke, 45
mitral stenosis, 54
mitral valve, 4, 6, 137
Mobitz type I second-degree heart block, 22-23, 191
Mobitz type II second-degree heart block, 22, 23, 178, 191–92
mouth to mouth breathing for CPR, 155, 156–57

MRI. *See* magnetic resonance imaging
myocardial infarction, 7, 27, 99, 112, 136, 192; family history of, 153
myocarditis, 138, 192

neurocardiogenic syncope, 53, 82, 178, 192, 196
niacin (nicotinic acid), 97, 99, 192
nil per os, 64, 65, 192
911, calling, 26, 46, 156, 166, 168
nitrates, 141
nitroglycerin, 97, 99
nonsteroidal anti-inflammatory drugs, 93, 192
normal sinus rhythm, 25, 59, 60
NPO. *See* nil per os
NSAIDs. *See* nonsteroidal anti-inflammatory drugs
nuclear cardiology studies, 8, 15
nuclear stress test, 63–64

oxygenation of blood, 5–6, 10

pacemakers, 4, 8, 105–8, 192; and AV junction ablation, 36; biventricular, 106, 114–16; for brady-cardia, 23, 44, 105; compared with ICDs, 109; dependence on, 36, 126; implantation of, 105–7; indications for, 105, 178; life of, 108, 124; permanent, 23, 36, 44, 178, 192; recovery after implantation of, 107–8; risks of, 107, 124; size of, 120
palpitations, 14, 26, 79, 117
paroxysmal supraventricular tachy-cardia, 25
PCI. *See* percutaneous coronary intervention
percutaneous coronary intervention, 9, 44, 74–76, 136, 138, 192. *See also* angioplasty; stents
percutaneous transluminal coronary angioplasty, 74
pericardial effusion, 192–93

26, 27–29, 43, 72, 94–96, 100,
196; antitachycardia pacing for,
109; and arrhythmogenic right
ventricular dysplasia, 71–72, 143;
automatic external defibrillator
for, 46, 160–62; catheter ablation
for, 89; and electrocardiogram, 62;
during electrophysiology study, 81;
and hypertrophic cardiomyopathy, 140; ICDs for, 109–13, 179;
medications for, 100; *torsades de
pointes*, 96, 193, 195
Viagra. *See* sildenafil

warfarin, 96, 98, 99–100, 196; and
atrial fibrillation / atrial flutter, 99;
stopping before stress test, 64
water pills. *See* diuretics
weight management, 153
Wolff-Parkinson-White syndrome,
30, 62, 196
WPW syndrome. *See* Wolff-
Parkinson-White syndrome

About the Author

Todd J. Cohen, M.D., F.A.C.C., F.H.R.S., is the Director of Electrophysiology, the Director of Advanced EP Technology and Innovations, and the Director of the Pacemaker-Arrhythmia Center at Winthrop University Hospital, Mineola, New York. He is an associate professor of medicine at the State University of New York at Stony Brook.

Dr. Cohen has published several articles in journals such as the *New England Journal of Medicine*, the *Journal of the American Medical Association*, *Circulation*, and the *Journal of the American College of Cardiology*. He has served for many years on the editorial boards of the *Journal of Invasive Cardiology* and *EP Lab Digest* (and is the emeritus editor-in-chief of the latter). He is also the author of the *Practical Electrophysiology* (second edition), a primer book for allied professionals, cardiology trainees, cardiologists, and electrophysiologists. He has served as principal investigator for multicenter studies such as MUSTT, SCD-HeFT, and the EnRhythm MRI trial. He has approximately twenty U.S. patents and has licensed and assigned inventions to several leading companies in the fields of resuscitation, electrophysiology, catheter ablation, and implantable devices. He is a member of the advisory board for the Sudden Cardiac Arrest Association, a not-for-profit patient advocacy charity.

Dr. Cohen is an avid collector of contemporary art and serves on the board of trustees of the Nassau County Museum of Art. He has been married to Jill for over two decades and has two children, eighteen-year-old Justin and fifteen-year-old Brittany.